The HISTORY
of the MANAGEMENT
# of PAIN

The HISTORY of the MANAGEMENT of PAIN

From early principles to present practice

Edited by Ronald D. Mann

The proceedings of a conference organised by
the SECTION OF THE HISTORY OF MEDICINE of
the ROYAL SOCIETY OF MEDICINE, London

The Parthenon Publishing Group
International Publishers in Science & Technology

Casterton Hall, Carnforth,
Lancs, LA6 2LA, U.K.

120 Mill Road, Park Ridge
New Jersey, U.S.A.

Published in the UK by
The Parthenon Publishing Group Limited
Casterton Hall, Carnforth,
Lancs, LA6 2LA, England

ISBN 1-85070-183-0

Published in the USA by
The Parthenon Publishing Group Inc.
120 Mill Road,
Park Ridge,
New Jersey 07656, USA

ISBN 0-940813-27-0

Photoset by Lonsdale Typesetting Services
Burton-in-Londale, Carnforth, Lancashire

Printed and bound in Great Britain
by Billing & Sons Limited, Worcester.

Contents

5

Contents

Contributors

Mrs Jennifer Beinart, MA
Research Officer
Wellcome Unit for the History of Medicine
University of Oxford
45–47 Banbury Road, Oxford OX2 6PE

Dr Doreen R. G. Browne, MSc, MB BS,
FFARCS, DCH, DObstRCOG
Consultant Anaesthetist
Royal Free Hospital
Pond Street, Hampstead, London NW3 2QG

Dr Patricia J. Flynn, FFARCSI, FFARCS
Senior Lecturer and Deputy Director
Anaesthetic Unit
The London Hospital Medical College
Turner Street, London E1 2AD

Dr Ashley Grossman, BA, BSc, MRCP
Senior Lecturer in Endocrinology
The Medical College of St Bartholomew's
Hospital
West Smithfield, London EC1A 7BE

Dr Helen King, BA, PhD
Trevelyan College
Elvet Hill Road, Durham
Co Durham DH1 3LN

Mr John R. Kirkup, MB BChir, FRCS,
DHMSA
Consultant Orthopaedic Surgeon
Royal United Hospital
Coombe Park, Bath,
Avon BA1 3NG

Dr Ronald D. Mann, MD, MRCP, MRCGP
Medical Assessor (Adverse Reactions)
Committee on Safety of Medicines;
Principal Medical Officer
Department of Health and Social Security
Market Towers, 1 Nine Elms Lane,
London SW8 5NQ

Prof. James P. Payne, MB ChB, FFARCS
Director
Research Department of Anaesthetics
The Royal College of Surgeons of England
35–43 Lincoln's Inn Fields
London WC2A 3PN

Dame Cicely Saunders, *DBE*, FRCP, FRCS
Chairman
St Christopher's Hospice
51–59 Lawrie Park Road,
Syndenham
London SE26 6DZ

Mrs Wendy D. Savage, MB BChir, FRCOG
Senior Lecturer in Obstetrics and
Gynaecology
The London Hospital (Mile End)
Bancroft Road,
London E1 4DG

Dr Malcolm Weller, MB BS, MRCPsych,
MBPsS
Consultant Psychiatrist
Friern Hospital
Friern Barnet Road
London N11 3PB

7

Preface

The inaugural meeting of what was intended to be called "The Section of Medical History and Literature" of the Royal Society of Medicine was held on Friday, 11 October, 1912, with Sir Francis Champneys, President of the Society, in the chair. The mover of the resolution which led to the formation of The Section of the History of Medicine was Professor Sir William Osler. The first ordinary meeting of the new Section was held on a Wednesday evening — 20 November, 1912 — when Osler was elected President of the Section. The Vice-Presidents included Sir T. Clifford Allbutt and the Honorary Secretaries were Raymond Crawfurd and D'Arcy Power.

Within a few months of the formation of the Section its activities became of great influence. Distinguished figures of medical history were made corresponding (honorary) members and the Section received many scholarly contributions of permanent value. In those years there were few places where such contributions could be published and it is of some importance that from the date of its formation, shortly before the outbreak of World War I, until 1939, and the outbreak of World War II, the Section of the History of Medicine was able to issue, as separately bound annual volumes, the published *Proceedings* of its meetings. These volumes contain vintage papers, many of which are of great academic merit, and it is a misfortune that it has been impossible to resume this series of publications. However, a substantial number of papers from the Section and its members have been published in the *Proceedings* and the *Journal of the Royal Society of Medicine*, whose successive editors have always been hospitable to the Section.

20 November, 1912, is almost exactly seventy-five years ago and it seemed appropriate to mark the 75th anniversary of the Section by holding a symposium on some subject of medical importance which could be considered from a historical point of view. It was also hoped to publish the proceedings so that they would be available for the Section meeting in November 1987. The subject of the management of pain was chosen as this has represented the abiding attempt of the profession of medicine throughout its long history.

Sir William Osler and his contemporaries knew, of course, the drugs of the early, mid, and late 19th century — respectively, the early alkaloids and glycosides, the early inhalational anaesthetics, and the early analgesics and barbiturates. Aspirin was introduced into medical practice in 1899, and barbitone, the lead drug of the great family of the barbiturates, was synthesised in 1903. Yet, up to 1910, scientific medicine recognised as specific remedies (that is, drugs which would attack the cause of an illness and not just allay its symptoms) only quinine in malaria, emetine in amoebic dysentery and mercury in syphilis. Ehrlich's introduction of his compound number 606, arsphenamine or "Salvarsan", took place in 1911 when it was first used in the treatment of human syphilis. Thus, this drug, the first fruit of the chemotherapeutic revolution which was to come, was available when the Section of the History of Medicine was founded. The 75-year history of the Section has, however, seen the discovery and development of almost the whole of the modern pharmacopoeia.

Even so, pain, in its many manifestations, still forces itself upon the attention of the contemporary physician and surgeon and the Section symposium of 1 April, 1987, considered several of its aspects. In order to remind us of the nature and extent of unrelieved acute pain, the symposium began with a talk on "Surgery before general anaesthesia" by Mr Kirkup, an orthopaedic surgeon from Bath. Doreen Browne, an anaesthetist, then spoke on "Ritual and pain", so reviewing the changes which altered mental and emotional states can make to the perception of pain. In order to look back at early means of relieving pain, Helen King, a classicist, then spoke on "The early anodynes".

10

Against this background, Patricia Flynn presented her joint paper with Professor James Payne on "The discovery and development of the contemporary anaesthetic agents".

The symposium then considered two modern issues connected with the management of pain, but reviewed from a historial point of view. The first of these studies was the present author's account of "The history of the non-steroidal anti-inflammatory agents". The second of these papers was Ashley Grossman's forward-looking discussion of "Opioid peptides and pain".

To look at the history of pain in special situations and at certain topics which we had selected as being of especial interest, the symposium ended with a group of four papers. Malcolm Weller, with a special eye on the social issues involved, reviewed the management of "The pain of psychosis". Dame Cicely Saunders presented a study of "The evolution of the hospices" — a paper which provides an insight into the experience of those who have contributed to this remarkable history. The growth of the pain clinics was then reviewed by Jennifer Beinart, whose book entitled *A History of the Nuffield Department of Anaesthetics, Oxford, 1937–1987*, from the Wellcome Unit at Oxford, has recently been published by the Oxford University Press. The meeting then closed with Wendy Savage's interesting and challenging view of "The management of obstetric pain".

It is satisfying to be able to preserve the proceedings of what proved to be a worthwhile meeting and I am sincerely grateful to Mr David Bloomer, Managing Director of The Parthenon Publishing Group, who has made publication possible. I also wish to note the good grace and gusto of the contributors called upon to support this symposium. The task of editing has been much assisted by my secretary, Mrs D. Noronha.

These proceedings, marking the 75th anniversary of the foundation of the Section of the History of Medicine, are dedicated to the memory of our foundation President, Sir William Osler.

Ronald D. Mann
Midhurst, Sussex

Foreword

"The conquest of pain remains, after all, the most important task, the main aim, and the crowning — though yet distant — achievement of every medical man, at the bedside, in the operating theatre, in the laboratory, on the battlefields, and wherever else mankind may suffer."

This was the concluding paragraph of the prize-winning Buckston Browne Prize Essay "The mental and physical effects of pain", which I had submitted to the Harveian Society of London on 1 October, 1948, and which was published by E & S Livingstone in 1949.

It will be readily understood, therefore, that I was delighted when Dr Ronald Mann, Secretary of the Section of the History of Medicine of the Royal Society of Medicine, suggested a whole-day symposium on the history of the management of pain, to be held jointly with the Section of Anaesthetics and the Scientific Research Section. It turned out to be a very successful meeting, held on Wednesday, 1 April, 1987, beginning at 10 a.m. and ending at 6 p.m. Ten speakers gave excellent papers, covering the subject through the ages, and were followed by lively discussion. We are very fortunate that the papers will be published in book form, edited by Dr Mann, and available at a reasonable cost. I wish it every success.

Cornelius Medvei
President, Section of the History of Medicine
Royal Society of Medicine, London

Chapter 1

Surgery before general anaesthesia

John Kirkup

Even if the prehistoric origin of surgery is unrecorded and obscure, it is clear that early man's instinctive reaction to serious injury played a fundamental role in the evolution of surgery. At the simplest level he would have sucked and squeezed a wounded finger to extract a thorn, exactly as we do today. At the other end of the scale, in the harsh environment which led to the survival of the fittest, man was subject to mortal injuries encountered in hunting animals, fighting his rivals and dealing with everyday domestic pursuits.

The patient as surgeon

Understandably, limbs severely savaged and trailing uselessly, or trapped under a fall of rock or a tree, would have prompted the desire to escape by lopping the limb free; initially, either the victim or a friend might have assumed the role of surgeon by using an axe. That this took place is suggested by records of animals escaping snares by self-amputation of the trapped limb; also by histories, such as that of a lumberjack in the Rocky Mountains, whose fate was recounted by Lord[1] in 1867 as follows. When standing on a log driving in wedges to split it, "... the man slipped, the wedge sprung instantly, and allowed the crack to close upon his foot ... shouting he knew to be useless, as there was no one within hail, and night was coming on, and he was well aware that the bitter cold of a northern winter must end his life long before any help could be reasonably anticipated — in his agony of mind and intensity of bodily suffering, with mad despair, the poor fellow seized the axe, and at a single chop severed his leg from the imprisoned foot." Sadly, although he was able to crawl to shelter, the incident proved fatal.

Further examples of desperation provoking autosurgery are not uncommon. In the 9th century Albucasis[2] related this account of a man's poisoned foot: "He had a blackening of the foot, with a burning like that of fire. The disease to begin with was in one toe, but it went on to involve the whole foot. When the man saw the disease spreading in the limb and felt the violent pain of burning, he hastened of his own accord to amputate it at the joint, and he got better." Albucasis then recorded that later the same man developed similar symptoms in a forefinger, and that these then spread to the rest of the hand. He urged Albucasis to cut it off, but the latter refused as he thought the man was too ill. He commented: "When he despaired of me he went back to his own country, I then heard that he had gone and cut off his whole hand, and got well. I narrate this story as help against this kind of malady when it occurs; and as guidance for you to take and act upon." Albucasis thought that he had failed the patient by ignoring self-preservatory instincts and instructions.

From the 15th and 16th centuries, Trolle[3] found accounts of self-inflicted Caesarean sections by nine mothers, of whom six survived. In the 17th century, Dean[4] observed the case of a man with a chronic urinary fistula, the consequence of an episode of acute urinary retention, which in desperation the victim relieved by passing a large pack needle per-urethram until he penetrated his bladder.

One can object, correctly, that these examples are not operations conducted by surgeons. Nonetheless, from a very remote period surgical-like instinctive responses by threatened victims probably encouraged the surgeon-class to repeat and refine life-saving procedures, as opportunity presented. Thus, almost certainly, self-inflicted operations contributed to the birth of emergency surgery.

Contemporary surgery without anaesthesia

Later, elective surgical procedures emerged, which were partly ritualistic in nature. These included circumcision, clitoridectomy, uvulectomy, finger amputation and trepanning. Indeed, these continue, often unaided by anaesthesia, as Meschig[5] observed in 1980 amongst certain tribes in Kenya where trepanning of the skull was being performed for persistent symptoms after head injuries. The operations, carried out with locally made tools, extended over many hours and often over several sessions. The authors concluded: "Africans are more capable of withstanding pain than Europeans, for they do not expect sympathy or pity from their fellows even if they complain." In the same year and the same part of Africa, Manni[6] gave a detailed account of uvulectomy, inappropriately undertaken for cough in young children, by a primitive technique without anaesthesia but, sadly, with many complications. Ritualistic circumcision, clitoridectomy and amputation of little fingers, especially in females, also continue in primitive societies without analgesia, though often during a state of mass hysteria.

Thus, there is past and present evidence to show that man can endure the pain of surgical incisions, either in circumstances of dire necessity when death is seen as a probability, or when there are strong ritualistic and tribal norms to be met, or when a mother is willing to risk all for an unborn child.

The search for pain relief

Nonetheless, attempts to avoid pain have been sought, at least since historical times. Among classical writers, Celsus and Theodoricus mention opium and hemlock as valuable agents taken before surgery but, although these are mentioned from time to time, little evidence of their use is recorded before the 11th century, when the soporific sponge evolved. In the 12th century Michael Scott wrote: "Take of opium, mandragora and henbane, equal parts. Pound and mix them with water. When you want to saw or cut a man, dip a rag in this and put it to his nostrils; he will soon sleep so deep that you may do as you wish." Sadly, he often slept too well. Opium or laudanum continued to be mentioned by surgeons, but principally as postoperative drugs. Bell[7] summed up the general attitude in 1796 by saying: "... it is best given after operations as it may cause vomiting if given before in sufficient dose to reduce pain." It is probable that imperfect standardisation of laudanum and opium, producing variable efficacy, reduced surgeons to this conservative approach.

Alçohol, frequently noted as a fortifier of resolution before an operation, is rarely recommended as an analgesic agent. In 1693 Moyle[8], a naval surgeon, writing of amputation, advised: "... give him a spoonful of cordial to stiffen him, then begin." Certainly, at sea it is often recorded that a tot of rum and a piece of leather to bite on were advantageous, as in the case of Horatio Nelson, whose right arm was amputated in 1797. Nevertheless, in his operation report, Nelson's surgeon, Thomas Eshelby, wrote: "Compound fracture of the right arm by a musket ball passing through a little above the elbow and artery divided. The arm was immediately amputated and opium afterwards given." Thus, again, the best available analgesic was reserved for postoperative care. Felkin[9], working in Uganda, in 1879 observed (Figure 1) a successful Caesarean section under banana wine inebriation. Similarly, Sands Cox[10] in 1842 recorded a disarticulation of the hip, without difficulty, by intoxicating the patient with half a bottle of port.

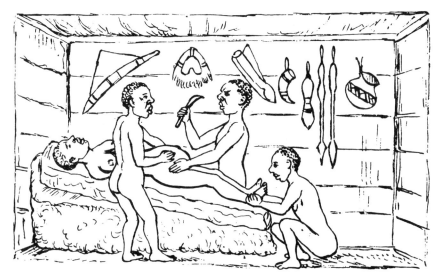

Figure 1 Caesarean section under banana wine inebriation in Uganda. Witnessed by Felkin in 1879

Other measures are noted by authors writing before anaesthetics were known. As early as 1363 Chauliac believed that a tight tourniquet produced a benumbing effect on the limb sufficient to ameliorate the pain of amputation. An extension of this approach was discussed in 1784 by Moore in his book *A Method of Preventing and Diminishing Pain in Several Operations of Surgery*, which introduced the application of specially made screw compressors (Figure 2) to stupefy individual nerves. However, after trials these devices were abandoned, as the pain of nerve compression was found objectionable.

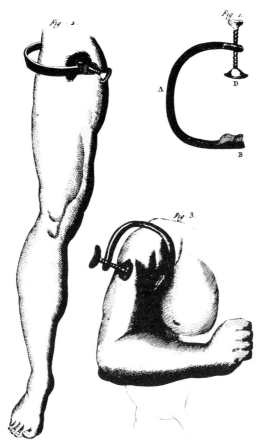

Figure 2 Nerve trunk compressor applied to sciatic and femoral nerves, and to axillary nerves. Introduced by Moore, 1784

Another remarkable instruction for amputation was to seat the patient in a firm chair whilst the surgeon knelt for a leg amputation and stood for an arm amputation — as shown in Figure 3. The seated posture would have encouraged fainting more readily, a condition of benefit to the patient. Surprisingly, there is little comment on the possibility of fainting, although Sir Charles Bell's drawings of a disarticulation at the shoulder (Figure 4) clearly demonstrate that the patient has fainted during the procedure.

Other surgeons recommended lower limb amputation with the patient positioned across a bed but sitting up. In 1739 Sharp[11] recommended a table exactly 30 inches in height to keep the surgeon upright and hence speed up the operation; even so, the patient was encouraged to sit (Figure 5).

Following observations on shattered limbs exposed to freezing conditions on the battlefield, deliberate refrigeration of limbs with ice was found to relieve the pain of amputation. Unhappily, sources of ice were limited before 1846, restricting the utility of this method. Judicious bleeding by venesection was said[12] to reduce apprehension

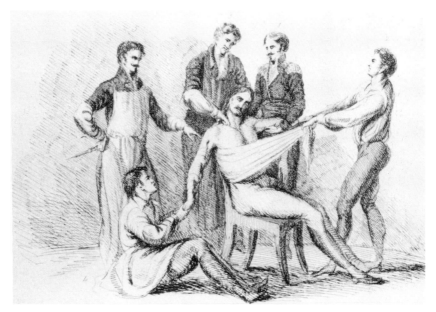

Figure 3   The seated posture for arm amputation. Drawn by C. Bell in 1821

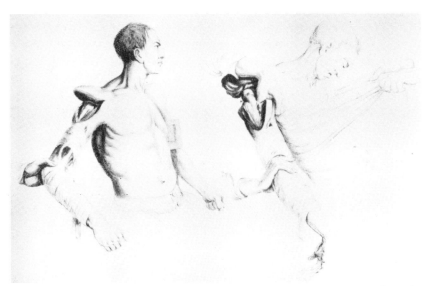

Figure 4 Disarticulation at the shoulder in the seated posture, causing the patient to faint. Drawn by C. Bell in 1821

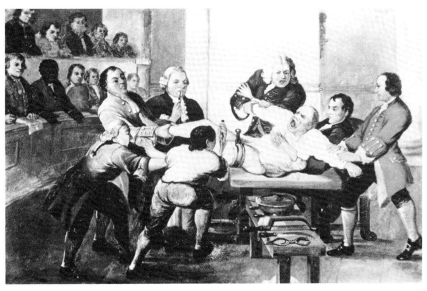

Figure 5 Lower leg amputation scene in old St Thomas's Hospital. Late 18th century, artist unknown

and, when combined with a hot bath and a tartar emetic, rendered the patient so low that the intense muscle spasm and severe pain associated with dislocation of the hip and shoulder could be overcome, so allowing manipulative reduction.

Exposure to stupefying gas also received notice. Davy[13] in 1800 suggested that nitrous oxide might be utilised in certain types of surgical operation and in 1824 Hickman[14] suggested the use of carbon dioxide. Regretfully, these ideas were not put to the test and, immediately prior to Morton's demonstration of ether anaesthesia in 1846, considerable publicity was given to the methods of mesmeric sleep or hypnosis by Elliotson, Esdaile and others.

Despite these innovations, none found favour with surgeons generally for, as Cooper[15] stated in 1822: "Modern practitioners have materially simplified all the chief operations in surgery, accomplished by better anatomical science, by devising less painful methods and by improving the construction of instruments." (Figure 6) Velpeau[16],

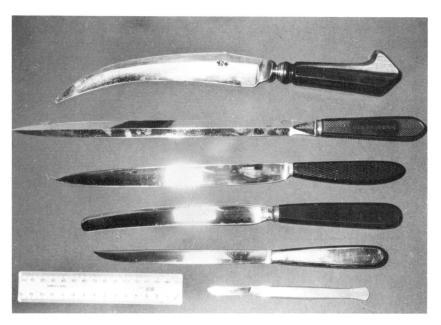

Figure 6 A selection of amputation knives from the mid-18th to the early 20th century, demonstrating gradual reduction in size and weight

commenting on the same topic in 1840, stated: "… these practices are a chimera, for it is better to have sharp scalpels, detailed knowledge and confidence, and the resignation of the patient"; but he added: "Immersing the instruments in hot water may reduce the pain." Cooper also thought that warming and oiling the instruments would help. Liston[17] emphasised the importance of speed and wrote in 1838: "The … parts should be divided by a single incision, rather than that the patient should be tormented … by a slow and tedious procedure, bit by bit." He also thought that, "… incisions from within outwards … give much less pain than those in the opposite direction." (Figure 7)

Thus, whilst pain was recognised as a significant factor restricting the nature of surgery that was possible, and perhaps the type of patient willing to submit to surgery, in general operations were tolerated with a fortitude that today appears mysterious and certainly astounding.

The following examples illustrate this, and also emphasise that it was the patient who insisted on relief and often demanded surgery. In the latter connection it is of interest to commence with an observation

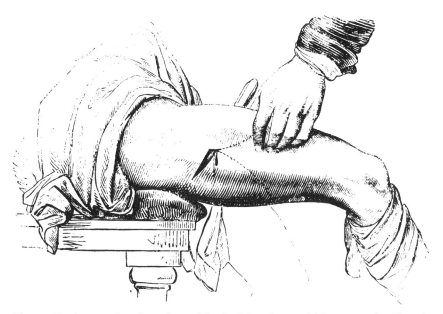

Figure 7 Amputation flaps formed by incision from within outwards. Liston's method in 1838

concerning a child, made by Ryder[18] in 1685. This involved a boy of nine who had been crushed by a cartwheel four years previously. He was confined to bed, emaciated, with eleven discharging fistulae. His heel was stuck to his buttock and his knee was dislocated. When Ryder, fearing to suggest amputation, said there was no possibility of cure, "The boy very heartily replied, he knew he should be well if I would cut off his thigh and if I would lend him a knife, he would cut it off himself." Persuaded by the child, he performed a thigh amputation. During this the boy did not cry while the knife or saw was used, but only during cautery of the vessels. Happily, the stump healed in six weeks and the boy gained weight and strength.

Similar pleading is noted by several authors, including Wiseman[19] in 1676. He reported a sailor who offered him a drink if only he would cut off a leg immediately, for, as was universally understood, men tolerated operations better when heated by battle action than the following day, when their courage cooled and their wounds became inflamed, tense and painful. Further, if men were put down into the ship's hold with a painful shattered limb, movement was extremely difficult and the hazard of being gnawed by rats was high. During the Peninsular War, Napier observed that after many battles two queues would form, one for arm and another for leg amputations. Often soldiers would see and certainly hear their comrades undergoing surgery, whilst the pile of discarded limbs was obvious. As Hennen[20] declared, and the men knew well, "It is better to live with three limbs than to die with four."

For the extraction of bladder calculi even greater resolution was needed. The condition was rarely an acute emergency, but rather a chronic illness which ground down the health of the patient, who often reached the point of passing urine every fifteen minutes, day and night. In such a situation even fearsome and dangerous surgery was accepted as the only practical source of relief. And, whilst death and urinary fistulae sometimes complicated lithotomy, there were many reported series with good results and low mortality. In 1662 Thomas Hollier, Surgeon for the Stone at St Thomas's Hospital, cut thirty without a death[21]. However, the following year he had four deaths. Samuel Pepys, cut by Hollier in 1658, had a stone the size of a tennis ball. It is said that Pepys was fortified for the occasion by a draught

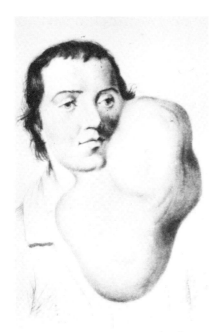

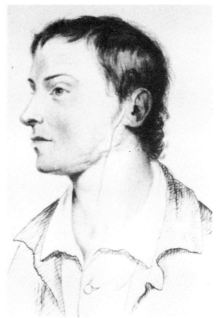

Figure 8 Massive salivary gland tumour present for sixteen years

Figure 9 The same patient after tumour excision by John Hunter in 1785. The procedure lasted twenty-five minutes.

containing liquorice, marshmallow, cinnamon, milk, rose-water and white of eggs. This was certainly no anodyne, but Pepys was ever grateful to Hollier and gave him an anniversary dinner thereafter. Unlike amputation, lithotomy required both a precise knowledge of anatomy and considerable manual dexterity and speed. Some of the greatest lithotomists extracted stones in under a minute. Cheselden's record was twenty-four seconds. Despite such feats, some patients refused operation and accepted a painful, lingering death.

Procedures involving tumour excision often took longer. John Hunter[22] recorded the removal, requiring twenty-five minutes, of a very large tumour from the face and neck of a man who did not cry out (Figures 8 and 9).

Brown[23] described a mastectomy for breast cancer, undertaken about 1839 by Syme. Although the duration is not stated, his account is revealing: "Alie stepped up on a seat, and laid herself on the table,

... the operation was at once begun; it was necessarily slow; and chloroform ... was then unknown. The surgeon did his work. The pale face showed its pain but was still and silent. It is over; she is dressed, steps down from the table, ... then turning to the surgeon and the students she curtseys, and in a low clear voice, begs their pardon if she has behaved ill. The students — all of us — wept like children."

During operations pain and fear were not the only problems for the patient, as indicated in a report describing plastic surgery on the nose of a syphilitic at St Thomas's Hospital in 1823[24]. Whilst the patient was lying supine the diseased nose was excised and a forehead pedicle flap fashioned to replace it. These procedures were completed by Mr Travers in about thirty minutes during which "... the patient was often obliged to raise himself from the table for the purpose of spitting out blood which got into his mouth ..."

The surgeon as patient

It is pertinent to remember that even in the pre-anaesthetic period surgeons themselves submitted to operations. The great Paré[25] instructed an apprentice to incise his leg to achieve reduction of a severe compound fracture. The first corrective osteotomy of the femur for flexion deformity at the knee was performed by Barton[26] on a young doctor in 1837; happily, the grateful patient was enabled to continue his practice. Another surgeon undergoing mid-thigh amputation graphically recorded his thoughts on the searing flash of overwhelming pain and anguish associated with the skin incision.

What then of the effect on the operating surgeon? Charles Bell[27] wrote: "When we thus consider the weight of responsibility, it is not surprising that so many shrink from the performance of the duties which belong to our Profession." He also wrote: "That the Surgeon, in order to do his duty, must be divested of the common feelings of Humanity, is a vulgar error." He concluded: "In truth, the anxiety of the Surgeon, before an important operation, is the greatest any man can suffer, ... the greatest Surgeon this country has produced, the celebrated Cheselden, was even in his later days, anxious to sickness, before the performance of a severe operation."

26

Anaesthesia spurned

Within a few months of the introduction of ether, South[28] wrote: "The year 1846 seems in a fair way to be known as the Annus Mirabilis of surgery." But he added: "... I have considerable doubt of the propriety of putting a patient into so unnatural condition as results from inhaling ether, which seems scarcely different from severe intoxication ...", and he was not alone in doubting the safety of anaesthesia. As late as 1858, Le Gros Clark[29] stated that he believed anaesthesia hazardous and left the option open to patients. Amazingly, many patients, swayed by his argument, permitted lithotomy without anaesthesia. However, the critics of anaesthesia were few and their doubts did not last long. Curiously, it was the patients themselves who were most conservative in accepting the benefits of ether and chloroform. Thus, Macormac[30], faced in 1870 with an old French soldier with bullets in both left shoulder and elbow, was asked to explore the wounds and remove the bullets and shattered bone without administering an anaesthetic, as the soldier wished to monitor the procedure and ensure amputation was not performed. And in the 1914–1918 war, Lériche[31], confronted by two wounded Cossacks, was forbidden by their officers to provide anaesthesia for men who felt no pain. With considerable repugnance, Lériche undertook two amputations during which, "Neither one man nor the other showed the least tremor, but turned a hand, or raised a leg when asked to do so, without showing even the slightest sign of momentary weakness, just as if under the most perfect local anaesthesia." He concluded that aspirin and anaesthesia had made men more susceptible to suffering, preventing them from acquiring toleration of pain and increasing the refinement of their senses, compared with their ancestors! The evidence presented in this essay suggests that these conjectures of Lériche are too facile.

Summary

We can conclude that:

(1) Under threat of death, self-operation by desperate victims suggested practical possibilities which encouraged surgical practitioners.

(2) Before 1846, the pain of operative surgery was borne for the most part with amazing fortitude.

(3) Whilst attempts to mitigate pain were sought, no method proved reliable before ether anaesthesia.

(4) Among western Europeans, pain was commonly accepted and endured as part of life's inevitable suffering; such acceptance was fostered by strong religious convictions.

(5) Today, in parts of Africa, patients adopt similar stoicism in the face of pain, in the knowledge that no sympathy can be expected from their peers.

(6) Finally, we must reflect that, whilst we know of the balm of anaesthesia, our ancestors did not. Indeed, such a miracle was not in their philosophy, whereas the instinct to survive often overcame their fear of pain. As John Bell inscribed on his title page for *The Operations of Surgery* in 1806, "Who would lose, for fear of pain, this intellectual being?"

References

1. Lord, J. K. (1867). *At Home in the Wilderness*. London: Hardwicke
2. Albucasis. In Spink, M. S. and Lewis, G. S. (eds) (1973). *On Surgery and Instruments*, pp 578–9. London: Wellcome
3. Trolle, D. (1982). *The History of Caesarian Section*, p. 29. Copenhagen: Acta Historica Scientiarum Naturalium
4. Dean, E. (1654). *Spadacrene Anglica, the English Spaw*, p. 39. York: Broad
5. Meschig, R. and Schadewaldt, H. (1981). Schädeloperationen in Kenia. *Dtsch. Med. Wschr.*, **106**, 157
6. Manni, J. J. (1986). Traditional uvulectomy in Africa. Presented at the XXX International Congress of the History of Medicine, September, Düsseldorf
7. Bell, B. (1796). *Cours Complet de Chirurgie*, 4th edn, Vol. VI, Ch. XLV. Paris: Barroiss
8. Moyle, J. (1693). *Chirurgus Marinus*, p. 52. London: Tracey
9. Felkin, R. W. (1884). Notes on labour in Central Africa. *Edin. Med. J.*, **29**, 922–30

10. Cox, S. (1845). *A Memoir on Amputation of the Thigh at the Hip Joint*. London: Reeve
11. Sharp, S. (1743). *A Treatise on the Operations of Surgery*, 4th edn, p. 215. London: Brotherton
12. Cooper, A. (1829). *A Treatise on Dislocations and Fractures of the Joints*, pp 24–5. London: Longman
13. Davy, Sir H. (1800). *Researches, Chemical and Philosophical, chiefly concerning Nitrous Oxide*. London: Johnson
14. Hickman, H. H. (1824). *A Letter on Suspended Animation,…* Ironbridge: Smith
15. Cooper, S. (1822). *A Dictionary of Practical Surgery*, 4th edn, p. 50. London: Longman
16. Velpeau, A. (1840). *Leçons Orales de Clinique Chirurgicale*, Vol. 1, p. 66. Paris: Baillière
17. Liston, R. (1838). *Practical Surgery*, 2nd edn, p. 7. London: Churchill
18. Ryder, H. (1685). *New Practical Observations in Surgery*. Observation XXIX. London: Partridge
19. Wiseman, R. (1676). *Severall Chirurgicall Treatises*, p. 420. London: Flesher
20. Hennen, J. (1820). *Principles of Military Surgery*, 2nd edn, p. 251. Edinburgh: Constable
21. Morris, C. G. R. (1979). A portrait of Thomas Hollier, Pepys's surgeon. *Ann. Roy. Coll. Surg. Engl.*, **61**, 224–9
22. Slaney, G. (1987). Hunterian Oration. Presented at the Royal College of Surgeons of England, February, London
23. Brown, J. (1859). *Horae Subsecivae*, pp 308–9. Edinburgh: Constable
24. Coulson, W. (1823). Hospital Reports: St Thomas's Hospital. *Lancet*, **I**, 436
25. Paré, A. (1678). *The Works*, p. 341. London: Clark
26. Barton, J. R. (1837). A new treatment for ankylosis. *Am. J. Med. Sci.*, *21*, 332–40
27. Bell, C. (1821). *Illustrations of the Great Operations of Surgery*, pp v–vii. London: Longman
28. South, J. F. (1847). In Chelius, J. M. *A System of Surgery*, Vol. II, p. 1007. London: Renshaw

29. Le Gros Clark, F. (1858). Quoted in *Med. Circ.*, **13**, 70
30. Macormac, W. (1939). In Lériche, R. *The Surgery of Pain*, p. 56. London: Baillière
31. Lériche, R. (1939). *The Surgery of Pain*, pp 2–3. London: Baillière

Chapter 2

Ritual and pain

Doreen R. G. Browne

This chapter tries to relate our knowledge of altered states of consciousness with an attempt to understand how certain ritualistic procedures can be undertaken without apparent pain. Ritual and pain may be considered together in two ways:

(1) Experiences associated with pain such as male and female initiation rites, childbirth, punishment and torture.
(2) Rituals associated with apparently traumatic procedures where pain perception appears to be changed.

It is this second aspect which will be considered here, with particular reference to people who walk on fire, performances by fakirs, hook-hanging and violent trance dances.

Fire-walking

This is a world-wide, cross-cultural phenomenon stretching back for centuries. Hopkins[1] related a story of two priests in India in about 1200 BC who walked through fire in order to determine who was the better Brahmin by not getting burned. Frazer[2] reported a wide selection of rituals involving fire. The earliest report he gave comes from the Greek geographer, Strabo, at about the time of Christ, who reported that priestesses walked unimpaired over glowing coals. It

31

was suggested that this may have been used either as a test of chastity or as a substitute for burning people. In another example, from Perasia, Frazer wrote that the priestesses' immunity from burning may be attributed to their inspiration and incarnation with the deity. Biblical reference to faith in the power of God to protect his followers against fire can be found in Isaiah[3]: "when thou walkest through fire, thou shalt not be burned". Among the members of the Church of God and Free Pentecostal Holiness Churches in the USA, immunity from being burned by fire is a trial of faith which was in vogue in the 1920s and still takes place occasionally today[4]. Fire-walking in the 20th century is practised in areas as widespread as North America, Siberia, Europe, Africa, India, Sri Lanka, Japan and Polynesia.

The Polynesian accounts describe rituals involving walking across hot stones or rocks, rather than coals. One of the earliest accounts appeared in 1893 and described walking through a "hot oven" made of heated stones[5]. An account of Europeans walking across the red-hot stones in this area was given by Gudgeon[6] in 1899. During this process one European got badly burned, which was said to be because "like Lot's wife, he looked behind him — a thing against the rules". Some of the earliest accounts showing scientific interest in this phenomenon came from Fiji where Fulton[7] considered that the immunity from burning was related to the slow radiation from the basaltic rocks, poor heat conduction, poor radiation and the cool nature of the feet which were only in momentary contact with the heated stones.

The first account of fire-walking in England appeared in the *British Medical Journal* in 1935 in an article by Price[8]. Two separate scientific demonstrations were given by Kuda Bux, a Kashmiri Indian. On each occasion he took four steps in four seconds to cross the trough of hot coals and showed no evidence of burning. Darling[9] wrote that having attended these demonstrations, he considered fire-walking to be a gymnastic feat. His calculations showed that the period of contact per impact with the hot coals was half a second and he considered this would not give enough time for blistering to occur. In 1936 Ernest Thomas[10] walked across red-hot embers in his threadbare socks, without "singeing, scorching and blistering". He attributed the immunity of fire-walkers from burning to the presence of ash, the cold legs and feet after preliminary bathing, the nature of the stones used, meditation and self-hypnosis. He considered that hypnosis itself would lower the temperature of the legs and protect them from blistering. It is of interest to note that the role of hypnosis in protecting against the inflammatory response to injury by burns is receiving some attention today by Dabney Ewin[11], a surgeon in New Orleans.

In 1971 another scientific account of fire-walking was given by Carlo Fonseka[12] in Sri Lanka, where he is Professor of Physiology at Colombo University. In a series of experiments he found that the length of time of contact of the feet with the hot embers was less than 0.6 seconds in those who were not burned. He also showed that there was no need for the participants to undergo any ritual deprivations beforehand in order to acquire protection from burning. Fonseka deduced from his experiments that the length of time of contact and state of the feet were critically important factors. These experiments met with heated opposition from the fire-walking devotees in Sri Lanka, as described by Wijeywardene[13].

This antagonism arose because fire-walking in Sri Lanka is looked upon as a supernatural phenomenon and the devotees claim that they do not get burned because divine aid protects them. Obeyesekere[14], writing in 1978, suggested that "fire-walking is both an act of faith and a test of faith". Those that get burned are being punished for lack of "bhakti" or for failure to fulfil the purification rituals. He said that many walk repeatedly in order to prove their faith. Others come to show gratitude for favours that the god Skanda has granted. Many of the devotees that walk the fire and perform other acts of penance have been ill or spirit possessed. Those who had been possessed considered that they had been transformed by these rituals into a vehicle for the deity. Fonseka[12] was challenged publicly about his findings by the President of the Fire-walkers and Kataragama Devotees, Sangamaya, who asked him whether a person would get burned if the contact time was over one minute. Fonseka replied: "If a person can keep his bare feet in continuous contact with glowing cinders having a temperature of 600–800 °F for over one minute without getting burned, then I will freely admit that the science I know cannot explain it." The debate over these experiments continues to the present day and has become a controversy concerning "Science versus Religion", "mind over matter" and "the power of God, not Science".

Recently, further studies have been performed on fire-walking, this time in Greece, Germany and England. In the period between 1978 and 1980 Wolfgang Larbig, a psychiatrist from Tübingen, and colleagues[15-17] monitored EEG recordings by telemetry while the participants walked across hot coals in experiments in Greece and Germany. Their findings showed the presence of large theta waves in the parietal regions of the brain in the beginners but not in the more experienced fire-walkers. Theta waves are shown in Figure 1.

In 1985 Hugh Bromiley, an American hypnotherapist, brought the "coal stroll"[18] to West London, claiming, "The mind can control pain and bodily responses and so I can introduce people to powers they never knew they possessed."[19] Members of the general public were invited to participate, paying £50 each for the evening. The first part of the evening involved a type of hypnotic state work-up during which the individuals wrote down on paper all their personal fears. These were then ritualistically burned in the leaping flames before the walk began. Immediately prior to the walk each participant stood in a cold wet muddy patch in front of the now glowing coals, chanting

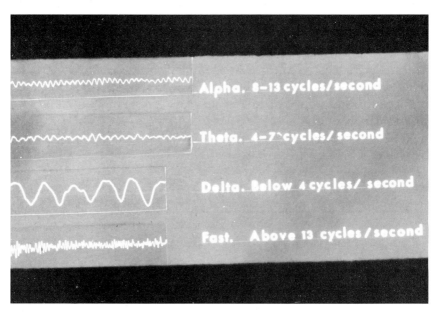

Figure 1 Patterns of electroencephalographic activity

"cool-wet-grass". When ready, each participant continued to chant these words and stare ahead while walking swiftly along the patch approximately 12 feet long. The majority of the people walked across relatively unscathed. However, one woman who did get burned had been observed to be walking across the hot coals more slowly than the rest and had seemed to be in quite a deep hypnotic trance. Towards the end of the walk she suddenly leapt off the coals and was immediately noted to have been burned. When asked why she thought she had got burned her reply was that her attention had been distracted by something and therefore the state of her mind was no longer protecting her. However, the more sceptical observers of the events felt that her trance-type state had allowed her to wander over the coals too slowly, thus giving time for her feet to burn; the pain of this had then jolted her out of her altered state of consciousness. The physical measurements made by the scientists present, including Professor Patrick Wall and Professor John Taylor, correlated with those made by Professor Carlo Fonseka in 1971 in Sri Lanka.

It seems clear from these scientific studies that people may walk the fire uninjured, provided they observe the principles of physics. Such an act needs courage and motivation, however, whether an individual is a scientist or a devotee. Indeed, many of the people who walked the fire in London claimed that it was the overcoming of the fear of walking across the glowing coals that provided the tremendous sense of exhilaration and achievement that had culminated in a successful fire-walk. The sharing of such an experience among a number of people who had been strangers before was a highly significant feature of this dramatic evening.

Fakir studies

During the time they were monitoring the fire-walkers in Germany, Wolfgang Larbig and colleagues[16, 17] were able to study a 48-year-old Mongolian fakir who had been working as a "pain artist" for many years. This fakir had suffered a painful illness during childhood and had discovered that he could stop his pain by fixing his gaze upon a distant point. He had then experimented with his mother's knitting needles and found that he could pierce his arms without pain. He

35

had elaborated his skills from then on. His performance was always preceded by several hours of concentrated meditation. Following this he could perform various manoeuvres without pain, such as inserting daggers through his neck, piercing his tongue with a sword and sticking needles through his arms. Larbig's study revealed some interesting findings. It was noted that throughout the whole procedure, lasting 20–30 minutes, the fakir would stare fixedly ahead and was observed not to blink for periods of up to five minutes. At the end of the performance there was an immediate and rapid return to a normal alert state of consciousness. Blood samples were taken thirty minutes before the start and thirty minutes after the conclusion of the performance, and samples of cerebro-spinal fluid were taken thirty and fifty minutes after the end. These samples showed evidence of increased catecholamines in the blood at the termination of the procedure. The cerebro-spinal fluid samples showed no evidence of endorphins. During the procedure it was noted that the automatic reflexes were increased, as was the skin inductance time. It was of particular interest that there was no evidence of pain resulting from the performer's own procedures but that he complained bitterly about needle pricks for venepuncture and discomfort from the inflated blood pressure cuff!! Electroencephalographic (EEG) recordings showed evidence of increased theta activity, especially in the parietal cortex. Similar EEG activity was found in members of a hook-hanging group of people Larbig studied in Sri Lanka.

Hook-hanging

Hook-hanging is another act of penance and religiosity known for centuries; and these rituals in Sri Lanka have also been discussed by Obeyeskere[20]. This phenomenon involves the spectacular performance of devotees being hung and swung from scaffolding, suspended by hooks through their flesh. Some of the earliest accounts of this ritual came from southern India. Thurston[21], quoting from a Government of Madras report in 1854, wrote that such a "cruel and revolting practice should be abolished, particularly as people have died as a result". Hocart[22], writing in 1927, described the ritual in Ceylon as either a trial by ordeal or a survival of a form of human sacrifice.

Obeyeskere suggested that such rituals are characteristic of an "arena culture", as the performances are always in public and are confined to special times and pilgrimage centres, like Kataragama[22]. Perera, an anthropologist in Sri Lanka, related in a personal communication that conditioning for this ritual takes place from childhood and involves increasing familiarity with procedures such as flesh piercing and needles being pushed through the cheeks and tongue before progress is made to the more dramatic rituals of hook-hanging without apparent pain. Rituals such as hook-hanging are not performed by laymen and, as each successful performance enhances the devotee's own ability to cope without pain, Perera claims a state of mind develops which the average person does not possess.

Like fire-walking, the ritual of hook-hanging has been a challenge for scientists as well as for philosophers and anthropologists. The points of scientific interest revolve around the lack of tearing of the flesh while the devotee is suspended, the relatively little bleeding and the apparent lack of pain. In March 1973 Fonseka[23] wrote an article which he called "The mystery of the hanging Kavadi". He hypothesised that the skin did not tear because the body weight was distributed uniformly between 8–12 hooks. He suggested that the minimal bleeding could be associated with skin tension and capillary vasoconstruction resulting from locally released agents. He concluded that the outstanding feature was the lack of pain throughout and that this phenomenon remained unexplained.

In the performance that I witnessed in 1983 it was noticeable that the participants stared fixedly ahead throughout most of the period; at no time were there any expressions of pain, including the periods of insertion of the hooks, the swinging itself, and the removal of the hooks. The equipment used is shown in Figure 2 and the actual episode of suspension in Figures 3 and 4.

It is interesting to note that the senior man appeared to be anxious during parts of his performance. When asked about this afterwards, he explained that he had not been concentrating properly, because he was distracted by looking round to see if the rest of the members of his troupe were fulfilling their roles correctly. All participants were fully alert throughout. At the end of each demonstration, the participant was lowered on to the table and the operators applied

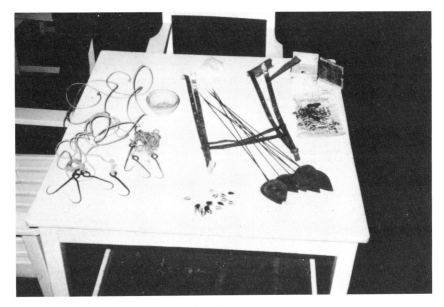

Figure 2   Apparatus used in hook-hanging

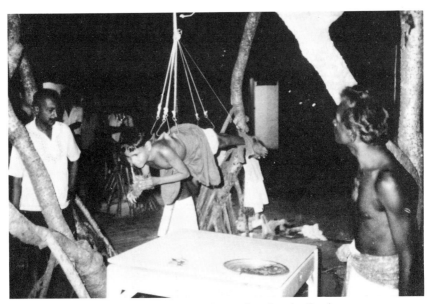

Figure 3   Hook-hanging by a young subject, showing the fixed gaze

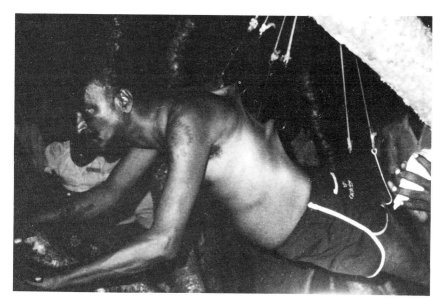

Figure 4 Hook-hanging by an older subject

firm manual pressure over the skin site of entry of each hook as it was removed. There was virtually no bleeding from the small holes left behind. The absence of pain was outstanding.

Larbig's EEG investigation of these people in the laboratory in Colombo in 1982 (described in a personal communication) showed theta wave activity present in all participants throughout the insertion of the hooks, the whole period of swinging and during removal. In summarising the significance of this theta activity in their various studies, Larbig and colleagues[17,24] suggested that it might appear as a correlate of a change of state of consciousness which serves to reduce anxiety and these waves may reflect some protective mechanism against pain.

The nature of pain

What, then, are the issues in this saga of dramatic "arena culture" performances? What is pain? The International Association for the Study of Pain (IASP) Subcommittee on Taxonomy in 1979[25] gave an official definition of pain as "an unpleasant sensory and emotional experience associated with actual or potential tissue damage or described in terms of such damage". Wyke[26] summarised some of the special aspects of pain as follows:

(1) Only the individual concerned can give an assessment of the pain he is feeling.
(2) There is no necessary correlation between the intensity of the emotional experience that is pain and the degree of tissue abnormality evoking it.
(3) Pain tolerance is more significant than pain threshold measurements as it is this component of tolerance which is so widely influenced by the individual, age, sex, race and cultural background.

Two classical studies have substantiated the theory of the effect of ethnic differences in response to pain. In 1952 Zborowski[27] studied 87 patients in the Veterans Hospital in Bronx, New York, who were men suffering from herniated discs and spinal lesions. He divided them into groups of Italians, Jews, "old" Americans and Irish. In 1965 similar groups of 60 housewives were studied in the laboratory by Sternbach and Tursky[28], who noted the responses of these women to electric shock stimulation. The results from both these studies showed that the Italians freely expressed their pain, that they derived immediate relief from therapy and that they had a lower level of pain tolerance. The Jews freely expressed their pain but its meaning and future implications were much more important than immediate relief. The Yankees, or "old" Americans, and the Irish were relatively undemonstrative in respect of their pain; they derived immediate relief from therapy but they preferred to suffer silently and alone. These responses may be summarised in a statement made by Hardy, Wolff and Goodell[29] who, in 1952, wrote: "The culture in which man finds himself becomes the conditioning influence in the formation of the individual reaction patterns to pain. A knowledge of group attitudes towards pain is extremely important to an understanding of the individual reaction."

It has been well known for many years that certain types of injury, such as war wounds and sports injuries, are characterised by an initial lack of pain. Beecher[30,31], in two papers in 1946 and 1956, discussed soldiers injured in the war at the Anzio beachhead. He found that about 66% of them were analgesic initially. He attributed this to a state of euphoria and relief arising from the knowledge that such wounds would enable them to escape from the danger zone. In contrast, Wall[32] in 1979 described soldiers who had to undergo amputation in the Yom Kippur War as being angry and resentful, in spite of showing a similar degree of immediate analgesia. Wall suggested that this immediate analgesia could be associated with the patients' attention being focused on fighting and escaping. Melzack, Wall and Ty[33] studied wounded civilians admitted to an Emergency Clinic in 1982 and found that 37% were analgesic initially, although their state of mind was one of worry.

In 1980 Fraioli and colleagues[34] produced evidence of the liberation of endorphins in vigorous exercise. In a double-blind study of long-distance runners, Janal and co-workers[35] have shown that these runners experience hypoalgesia with a "runner's high" and that these effects are associated with an increase in beta-endorphin concentra-tions which are inhibited by naloxone (an opiate antagonist). A very recent paper by Dale and his associates[36] has suggested that these com-pounds may play a major role in the collapse of "fun run" or marathon runners. Henry[37] discussed the possible role of endorphins in ecstatic trance-type rituals. Crapanzano[38], in a study of the Hamadsha in Morocco, described a vivid ritual comprising violent ecstatic dancing, hyperventilation, and special dance rhythms associated with the slashing of the head using a knife. All the participants appeared to be totally unaware of their injuries. The role of endorphins in such rituals, however, has yet to be scientifically defined.

The next question to be clarified in the rituals described concerns the nature of the state of consciousness of the individual concerned. Is the individual in an altered state and if so what is its nature? Hypnotic states will be considered first.

Hypno-anaesthesia in India was described in a classic study by Esdaile[39]. In 1974, Hilgard[40] discussed his theory of multiple cognitive controls in hypnotic analgesic states using the "hidden observer" technique. In this paper Hilgard demonstrated that the hypnotised subject would report verbally that his arm immersed in ice-cold water was pain-free. However, the opposite hand (freed from hypnotic influence) would write and assess the pain on the same scale as in the normal awake state. In some way there seemed to be distortion of the perception of pain in the hypnotic analgesic state. However, once the discovery of endorphins had been made it was interesting to see if they had any role to play in hypnotic analgesia. In 1975 Goldstein and Hilgard[41] found that naloxone did not reverse the hypnotic analgesia provided to protect against pain from an ischaemic tourniquet. It was therefore concluded that hypnotic analgesia was not the result of endogenous opiates and so must result from some different neurological mechanism. In 1976 Banyai and Hilgard[42] and in 1980 Banyai[43] used awake, alert focusing induction techniques as a means of inducing successful hypnotic states. These methods are different from the more classical relaxation techniques. Orne[44] in 1980 suggested that during the induction of hypnosis there is a refocusing of the individual's attention and it is this which alters important cognitive processes.

In 1971 Oatman[45] had performed some experiments on cats, which showed that by focusing attention on visual stimuli the appreciation of auditory stimuli monitored by evoked potentials in the brain could be inhibited during that explicit period. In this context it is of interest that modern methods of testing hearing in very small children and babies, using evoked potentials, require that the individual is anaesthetised in order to ensure that the auditory stimuli are not inhibited from reaching the brain by distractions which could occur if he were awake.

The role of attention in hypnosis and meditation has been described and discussed by various writers. Anand and his co-workers[46] and Banquet[47] described some fascinating EEG studies they performed on yogis practising meditation. Yogis engaged in Samadhi meditation claim they are oblivious to external and internal environmental stimuli during the period of meditation. In the Anand study four yogis had EEG recordings before and during meditation. Two of them were exposed to stimuli in the form of loud noise, hot rods, vibration and lights. The other two were exposed to hand immersion in water at 4 °C for 45–55 minutes. Under normal non-meditating conditions, the alpha rhythms of the brain would be blocked by such strong stimuli. During the period of meditation, in all types of experiment all the yogis showed persistent increased alpha activity which was not blocked by any of the stimuli. The authors concluded that meditating individuals appear to be able to block afferent impulses from the reticular activating system of the brain ever reaching the cortex and so remain in persistent alpha activity.

Banquet's study involved spectral analysis of the EEG in twelve yogis practising transcendental meditation (TM) using a "mantra" and twelve matched controls practising relaxation. All subjects were exposed to flashing lights and auditory clicks as stimuli. At the beginning, some of the controls showed alpha activity which could be blocked by stimuli. In a more stable sleepy state there was a mixed picture of alpha and beta activity in four of the controls and alpha and delta activity in four of the others. The remaining four did not develop a stable alpha rhythm. In contrast, the meditators all showed positive alpha activity at the beginning and this was not blocked by stimuli. As the meditators stabilised, the alpha activity changed to theta waves. In stage II meditation there were continuous unmixed trains of theta activity, which were only blocked for a second when the stimuli were applied, converting immediately back to the theta pattern. At the end of the procedure theta activity was still seen in some of the yogis, even with their eyes open in the postmeditation period. In his conclusion Banquet suggests that the EEG recordings from meditators practising TM distinguish the meditative state from other states of consciousness, including auto-suggestion and hypnosis. Davidson and Goleman[48] hypothesise that during intense concentration in meditation incoming sensory information may be blocked below the level of the cortex, while in hypnosis the sensory experience of the pain remains the same but the experience of the suffering is reduced, as shown by the Hilgard experiment.

In a lecture to the British Society of Medical and Dental Hypnosis at the Royal Society of Medicine in 1982, Wyke[49] discussed "The neurophysiology of hypnosis". He suggested that the descending neural tracts from the frontal cortex to the caudal end of the reticular system may be involved in the hypnotic process and that the transmitters have not yet been identified. In 1986 Wall[50] addressed the same society on "The neural mechanisms of pain-free states". In the discussion following his lecture the Hadfield experiments[51] and the Moody reports[52,53] were discussed. In the Hadfield experiments in 1917 a seaman was studied who was undergoing hypnotherapy for symptoms of shellshock. During the procedure a finger was placed on his arm and the patient was told that he was being touched by a red-hot iron. The arm was immediately withdrawn in evident pain. It was then suggested, still under hypnosis, that a blister would form. The patient was woken up. Half an hour later he returned complaining of a painful reddened area on the arm with a blister developing and asked if anything had happened while he had been under hypnosis. The Moody reports concern bodily changes during abreaction. Several cases were described and two are of particular interest. One case report concerns the appearance of deep wheal-like rope marks on the forearms of a patient during the abreaction of an accident that had occurred ten years previously. The second case concerns the appearance of cutting-whip marks on the back of the hands of a patient who had been inflicted with these insults in early life. Wall ended the meeting with the words: "The challenge in all of this is to try to explain a highly organised local phenomenon. If claims that one arm can be made hot and the other cold under the influence of the mind could be supported scientifically then this is revolutionary and the whole concept of pain pathways as we know them will have to be rethought."

At the beginning of his Buckston-Browne essay in 1948, Dr Medvei[54] commented that pain had been studied extensively during the preceding forty years but that tremendous gaps remained. It is now nearly "forty years on" and in spite of the major breakthroughs that have occurred in research in this subject, such as Melzack and Wall's "gate theory of pain" and the discovery of the endogenous opiates, it seems that a number of chasms still remain. In 1952, Zborowski[27] said that "... physiological phenomena can become institutions regulated by cultural and social norms, thus fulfilling not only biological functions but social and cultural ones as well". Perhaps during the next forty years the experts will look further at the other side of this cross-cultural coin in order to unravel "the mystery of analgesia".

Acknowledgements

I am deeply indebted to the following:

Dr Wolfgang Larbig (Tübingen, West Germany),
Professor Ioan Lewis (London School of Economics, London),
Dr Peter Nathan (The National Hospital for Nervous Diseases, Queen
    Square, London), now retired;
Professor Patrick Wall (University College Hospital, London),
Professor Barry Wyke (Royal College of Surgeons, London), now
    retired;
Susan Siklawi for secretarial help;
Pauline Summers (Librarian, Royal Free Hospital);
Medical Illustration Department, Royal Free Hospital; and
Nihal Jayaweera, Sri Lanka Fire-walkers Troupe, Colombo, 1983.

References

1. Hopkins, E. (1913). *Encyclopaedia of Religion and Ethics*, Vol. 6, pp 30–1. New York: Scribners
2. Frazer, J. (1911–1915). *The Golden Bough: A Study of Magic and Religion*, 3rd edn, Vol. V, Bk 1, Ch. 5, p. 115, and Vol. V, Bk 1, Ch. 6, p. 169. London: Macmillan & Co.
3. Isaiah 43:2. *The Bible*
4. Kane, S. M. (1982). Holiness ritual and fire handling. *Ethos*, **10**, No. 4, 369–84
5. Henry, T. (1893). TE UMU-TI. A Raiatean ceremony. *J. Polynesian Soc.*, **2**, 105–8
6. Gudgeon, C. (1899). TE UMU-TI or fire-walking ceremony. *J. Polynesian Soc.*, **8**, 58–60
7. Fulton, R. (1902). An account of the Fiji firewalking ceremony or Vilavilairevo, with a probable explanation of the mystery. *Trans. N. Z. Inst.*, **XXXV**, 187–201
8. Price, H. (1935). Fire walking experiments: report on Kuda Bux's demonstration. *Br. Med. J.*, **2**, 586
9. Darling, C. R. (1935). Fire-walking (correspondence). *Nature*, 28 September, 521
10. Thomas, E. S. (1936). Fire-walking. *Nature*, 8 February, 213–5

11. Ewin, D. M. (1979). Hypnosis in burn therapy. In Burrows, G. D., Collinson, D. R. and Dennerstein, L. (eds) *Hypnosis*, pp 269–75. Elsevier/North Holland Biomedical Press

12. Fonseka, C. (1971). Fire-walking: a scientific investigation. *Ceylon Med. J.*, June 1971, 104–9

13. Wijeywardene, G. (1979). Fire-walking and the scepticism of Varro. *Canberra Anthropology*, **2**, 114–33

14. Obeyesekere, G. (1978). The fire-walkers of Kataragama: the rise of Bhakti religiosity in Buddhist Sri Lanka. *J. Asian Stud.*, **37**, No. 3, 463–6

15. Larbig, W., Lutzenberger, W., Elbert, T., Rochstroh, B. and Birbaumer, N. (1981). EEG and slow cortical potentials related to laboratory pain and EEG correlates of pain during firewalking in Greece. *Pain*, **Suppl. 1**, S57

16. Larbig, W., Haag, G. and Birbaumer, N. (1981). Pain regulation and psychosomatics: Preliminary experiments and field studies on fire-walkers. In Zander, W. (ed.) *Experimentelle Forschungsergebnisse in der psychosomatischen Medizin*, pp 59–68. Göttingen: Vandenhoeck and Ruprecht

17. Larbig, W. (1982). *Schmerz. Grundlagen — Forschung — Therapie*, pp 190–9, 269. Stuttgart, Berlin, Cologne and Mainz: Verlag W. Kohlhammer

18. Inglis, B. (1985). Through the heat barrier. *The Guardian*, 5 June 1986

19. Thynne, J. (1985). Bromiley quoted in Hot foot shuffle. *The Sunday Times*, 16 June 1985, p. 36

20. Obeyeskere, G. (1981). *Medusa's Hair*, pp 142–9. London: The University of Chicago Press Ltd

21. Thurston, E. (1854). *Ethnographic Notes in Southern India*, pp 471–501. Madras: The Superintendent, Government Press

22. Hocart, A. M. (1927). Ceylon: Religion. Tukkam. *Man*, **110**, September, 161–2

23. Fonseka, C. (1973). The mystery of the hanging Kavadi. *The Nation*, 16 March

24. Larbig, W., Elbert, T., Lutzenberger, W., Rockstroh, B., Schnerr, G. and Birbaumer, N. (1982). EEG and slow brain potentials during anticipation and control of painful stimulation.

Electroenceph. Clin. Neurophysiol., **53**, 298–309

25. Mersky, H., Bonica, J. J. *et al.* (1979). Pain terms: A list with definitions and notes on usage. Recommended by the IASP Subcommittee on Taxonomy. *Pain*, **6**, 249–52

26. Wyke, B. D. (1981). Neurological aspects of pain therapy: A review of some current concepts. In Swerdlow, M. (ed.) *The Therapy of Pain*, pp 1–30. Lancaster: MPT Press Ltd

27. Zborowski, M. (1952). Cultural components in responses to pain. *J. Soc. Issues*, **8**, 17–30

28. Sternbach, R. A. and Tursky, B. (1965). Ethnic differences among housewives in psychophysical and skin potential responses to electric shock. *Psychophysiology*, **1**, No. 3, 241–6

29. Hardy, J. D., Wolff, H. G. and Goodell, H. (1952). *Reaction to Pain. Pain Sensations and Reactions*, pp 261–306. Baltimore: Williams & Wilkins Co.

30. Beecher, H. K. (1946). Pain in wounded men in battle. *Ann. Surg.*, **123**, 96–105

31. Beecher, H. K. (1956). Relationship of significance of wound to pain experienced. *J. Am. Med. Assoc.*, **161**, No. 17, 1609–13

32. Wall, P. D. (1979). On the relation of injury to pain. The John J. Bonica Lecture. *Pain*, **6**, 253–64

33. Melzack, R., Wall, P. D. and Ty, T. C. (1982). Acute pain in an Emergency Clinic: Latency on onset and descriptor patterns related to different injuries. *Pain*, **14**, 33–43

34. Fraioli, F., Moretti, C., Paolucci, D., Alicicco, F., Crescenzi, F. and Fortunio, G. (1980). Physical exercise stimulates marked concomitant release of β-endorphin and adrenocorticotropic hormone (ACTH) in peripheral blood in man. *Experientia*, **36**, 987–9

35. Janal, M. N., Cort, E. W. D., Clark, W. C. and Glusman, M. (1984). Pain sensitivity and plasma endocrine levels in man following long-distance running: effects of naloxone. *Pain*, **19**, 13–25

36. Dale, G., Fleetwood, J. A., Weddell, A. and Ellis, R. D. (1987). β endorphin: A factor in "fun run" collapse? *Br. Med. J.*, **294**, 1004

37. Henry, J. L. (1981). Circulating opioids: possible physiological roles in central nervous function. *Neurosci. Behav. Rev.*, **6**, No. 3, 229–45

38. Crapanzano, V. (1973). *The Hamadsha: A Study in Moroccan Ethnopsychiatry*, pp 185–211 and 231–5. London: University of California Press Ltd

39. Esdaile, J. (1846). *Mesmerism in India, and its Practical Application in Surgery and Medicine*. London: Longman, Brown, Green and Longmans

40. Hilgard, E. R. (1974). Towards a neo–dissociation theory: multiple cognitive controls in human functioning. *Perspec. Biol. Med.*, **17**, No. 3, 301–16

41. Goldstein, A. and Hilgard, E. R. (1975). Failure of the opiate antagonist Naloxone to modify hypnotic analgesia. *Proc. Nat. Acad. Sci.*, **12**, No. 6, 2041–3

42. Banyai, E. I. and Hilgard, E. R. (1976). A comparison of active-alert hypnotic induction with traditional relaxation induction. *J. Abnormal Psychol.*, **85**, No. 2, 218–24

43. Banyai, E. I. (1980). A new way to induce a hypnotic-like altered state of consciousness: active-alert induction. Problems of the regulation of activity. *Proceedings of the 4th Meeting of Psychologists from the Danubian Countries*, pp 261–73. Budapest: Akademiai Kiado

44. Orne, M. T. (1980). Hypnotic control of pain: Towards a clarification of the different psychological processes involved. In Bonica, J. J. (ed.) *Pain*, pp 155–72. New York: Raven Press

45. Oatman, L. C. (1971). Role of visual attention on auditory evoked potentials in unanesthetized cats. *Exp. Neurol.*, **32**, 341–56

46. Anand, B. K., Chhina, G. S. and Singh, B. (1961). Some aspects of electroencephalographic studies in Yogis. *Electroenceph. Clin. Neurophysiol.*, **13**, 453–6

47. Banquet, J. P. (1973). Spectral analysis of the EEG in meditation. *Electroenceph. Clin. Neurophysiol.*, **35**, 143–51

48. Davidson, R. J. and Goleman, D. J. (1977). The role of attention in meditation and hypnosis: a psychobiological perspective on transformations of consciousness. *Int. J. Clin. Exp. Hypnosis*, **XV**, No. 4, 291–308

49. Wyke, B. (1982). Neurophysiology of hypnosis. Lecture given to the Section of Medical and Dental Hypnosis, Royal Society of Medicine, 4 October 1982

50. Wall, P. D. (1986). The neural mechanisms of pain-free states. Lecture given to the Section of Medical and Dental Hypnosis, Royal Society of Medicine, 2 June 1986
51. Hadfield, A. (1917). The influence of hypnotic suggestion on inflammatory conditions. *Lancet*, **2**, 678–9
52. Moody, R. L. (1946). Bodily changes during abreaction. *Lancet*, 28 December, 934–5
53. Moody, R. L. (1948). Bodily changes during abreaction. *Lancet*, 19 June, 964
54. Medvei, V. C. (1948). *The Mental and Physical Effects of Pain*. Buckston Browne Prize Essay, Harveian Society of London, pp 5–59. Edinburgh: E. & S. Livingstone Ltd

Chapter 3

The early anodynes:
pain in the ancient world

Helen King

Any discussion of ancient drug therapy must begin with a number of caveats. It is certainly possible to find out which plant, animal and mineral substances were used in any particular medical context — in this case, as painkillers — but it is very difficult to assess the precise effects of any given substance. In an important recent study of the *Materia Medica* of Dioscorides, a work which dates to around 65 AD and covers over 1000 substances, John Riddle[1] issues the following warning: "If one searches the historical documents of medicine to find those drugs which appear in our modern medical guides, we distort the record." I would go further, and pose this question: can we simply search the ancient literature for the use of anodynes, or does the concept of "anodyne" differ from our own in ways so subtle yet significant that any such quest will fail to do justice to the historical material we study? How do we assess a remedy which was used for many hundreds of years, but which in terms of our current understanding is entirely ineffective? How do we match a modern drug use to an ancient drug?

Before we tackle such complex questions as these, there are many more obvious difficulties which stand in the way of an analysis of any part of the ancient pharmacopoeia. For example, most ancient medical texts do not give the quantities to be administered. This is not because the authors thought quantities unimportant since, as Riddle[2] points out for Dioscorides, quantities were more likely to be given when the substance in question was highly toxic. In general, however, medicine was supposed to be something learned from experience as well as from instruction, so that the practitioner would gradually learn how to weigh up all the variables both on the side of the patient — his or her age, constitution, how serious the condition — and on the side of the drug — how it had been prepared, how long ago it was harvested, and similar factors. With so many variables to be considered, no handbook could guarantee the best dosage.

Even when quantities are given, we cannot necessarily use this information to assess the efficacy of an ancient remedy, because we may not know whether the methods of harvesting and preparation of the materials for drugs were the same as now, nor indeed whether the chemical make-up of the plants was the same as that which we find today[3,4]. Attempts to match a modern plant to an ancient description or illustration may themselves prove inconclusive.

Another difficulty arises with the site of administration, which is just as important as the choice of drug. A plant may be employed which we now know to have certain chemical properties, but this does not mean that the ancient world used it in the best possible way. Garlic may have antibacterial qualities, but these will not be effective if it is worn around the neck by a patient with a stomach disorder; Hopkins[5] has pointed out that assessing the efficacy of contraceptive substances used in the Roman Empire is further complicated by the fact that individuals were apparently using several substances at once. A related point which should always be remembered is that ancient ideas about anatomy were often very different from our own, and this influenced the use of drugs. Such central discoveries as the circulation of the blood were many centuries away. When reading ancient texts, similarities in vocabulary should not lull us into a false sense of familiarity. The word "diaphragm" is a Greek word, but to the Greeks it — rather than the heart — often signified the seat of the emotions. Some groups in the ancient world saw the liver as the governing organ of the body; others gave this role to the heart[6]. Using an example from my own specialism, early Greek gynaecology, it was widely believed that women were basically hollow tubes with a "mouth" at each end, and that the womb could move around the body causing symptoms of many kinds. In this ethno-anatomy, epistaxis was the result of menstrual blood taking the route up the tube rather than down it, and applying remedies to either end of the tube would affect the womb[7]. We of course have a similar idea, that substances taken orally affect uterine function, but support it with a rather different rationale.

Our judgement of the efficacy of ancient ingredients is additionally complicated by the placebo factor. It is possible for us to give rational explanations for many items in the pharmacopoeia, but we cannot know, for the reasons already stated, whether their efficacy was due to entirely different considerations. Cantharid beetle pessaries feature in the Hippocratic gynaecological pharmacopoeia, and they would have an irritant and purgative effect; wild cucumbers are used as a purge, and they would have a laxative effect; urine is used in many recipes, and has antiseptic qualities; rubbing animal fat or oil on to sore skin would ease it. However, we cannot always reconstruct the reason why a substance was used in a particular context, and it is perfectly possible that a physician was doing the right thing for the wrong reason. Shape, colour, smell or a myth associating substance and symptom may have been more important to many early doctors and patients than chemical constituents. Thus, for many recipes it is impossible to judge, on the basis of the information given, whether the constituents would work, and in many cases the presence of items in the ancient pharmacopeia "clearly owes more to the symbolic associations of the substances in question than to their objective efficacy"[4,8]. For example, parts of male, virile animals — the penis of a stag, bull's bile — are credited with power. This does not mean that such substances should be dismissed as ineffective; the doctor and the patient apparently believed that they would work, and any efficacy depended on this belief.

A further important point influencing any assessment of ancient drug use is that the ritual of prescribing or administering the drug—in our culture, the white coat and the prescription pad — can affect its efficacy. In the ancient medical tradition words were very important; practitioners were expected to present their theories and explanations fluently, either in the context of a public debate with a rival, or in the more private context of a bedside consultation when the client — or potential client — needed to be persuaded of the healer's skills. Actions too were important in treatment, so that many therapies involved an element of dramatic display. Some were such good theatre that they would be carried out in public. For example, in a famous Greek text called *On Joints*, probably of the 4th century BC, a writer condemns those who practise the spectacular therapy of public succussion on a ladder, in which the patient is tied to a ladder and violently shaken. This could be done for many reasons; for example, to reduce a fracture, for prolapse of the womb or to induce labour. It is acknowledged to be dangerous but is continued because of its power to impress "the crowds"; even the writer who condemns it admits that sometimes it is very useful.

In such public therapies, the patient's illness is acknowledged and displayed to the onlookers; there is no trace here of the idea that one should keep one's ill-health to oneself. The cure, too, is displayed, and on its success or failure depends the future employment of the physician. But why would anyone willingly submit himself or herself to such a therapy in the first place? Ancient doctors were aware of the importance of trust, and tried to gain it by their appearance — clothing, demeanour and even perfume — as well as by their bedside manner, ideally calm, sympathetic but firm. Many texts discuss how to achieve this ideal, and it is possible that the appearance of the ideal doctor was as effective in announcing his identity and credentials as the white coat or dark suit of modern medical practitioners are today. Once the patient was put in the right frame of mind by the appearance and behaviour of the physician, and was persuaded by words and actions of the certainty of a cure, how can we hope to distinguish the efficacy of the drug from the efficacy of the context in which it was given?

With such caveats as these always in mind, I would now like to look briefly at the kinds of substance used to relieve pain in the ancient world, and then to look more closely at ancient Greek ideas on what pain is and how it should be handled.

The ancient world was acquainted with a number of anodynes known today. The Hippocratic text *Affections* mentions a lost work called *On Drugs* which apparently listed painkilling drugs: "To those suffering from these pains, one gives the *pharmaka* listed in *On Drugs* as those which stop pain" (*Affections* 15/L 6.224). Three types of henbane (black, yellow and white; Greek *hyoskuamos*), which contains hyoscyamine alkaloids, were known (e.g. Dioscorides 4.68) and were used as an anodyne in topical applications. A number of other plants containing tropane alkaloids — hyoscyamine, atropine and scopolamine — are also listed by Dioscorides[9]. These include belladonna (*strychnos manikos*), black nightshade (*strychnos*) and mandrake (*mandragoras*).

A point worth making here is that the Greek *pharmakon* means both the healing drug, and poison, something particularly important where the tropane alkaloids are concerned. Henbane is seen as sufficiently dangerous that Dioscorides gives a standard dosage for it; however, for opium he does not. This seems surprising but Riddle[10] suggests that, because Dioscorides knew that the time of harvesting was particularly important in determining the efficacy of opium, he would expect the physician to bear that in mind when prescribing quantities. Galen had a different attitude to the dangerous drugs; he warned that detailed descriptions of poisonous plants only gave the unscrupulous information which could endanger life[11]. Theophrastus, writing in the 3rd century BC, says that two drachms of *strychnos manikos* produce delusions, three insanity, and four death; even allowing for the difficulties of comparing wet and dry measures, this suggests that the use of these drugs had progressed somewhat since a Hippocratic writer had recommended a quarter of a pint of this drug daily, as a painkiller[12].

The opium poppy originated in Asia Minor, and opium has been used from very ancient times to produce sleep; it is described in the 3rd century BC. Dioscorides distinguishes between the juice from the capsules, *opos*, from which we derive the name opium, and *mekonion*, the extract of the whole plant. Opium is an important ingredient in many ancient remedies; in particular, it has been suggested that it is the active constituent of the cure-all called theriac, a medicine with a vast number of ingredients which varied according to the particular physician making it up and according to the availability of certain substances[13]. It was supposed to cure snakebite, headache, vertigo, deafness, apoplexy, epilepsy, asthma, colic, jaundice, the stone, fever, and many other conditions.

An insight into how the Greeks and Romans thought about drug action is given by Dioscorides' classification of the plants containing tropane alkaloids as "cooling"; some, like wild lettuce (*agria thridax*), which contains hyoscyamine, are thought to be a little less cooling than the others. By this Dioscorides appears to mean that they slow down the vital functions[14]. In ancient thought, life is often seen as "warm", death "cold", and ageing therefore as a process of cooling down and drying out[15].

Concentrating on the drugs known to be effective painkillers today may, however, be misleading. A treatment of pain which is perhaps more typical is the use of fomentations. Chapter 7 of the Hippocratic treatise called *Regimen in Acute Diseases* (L 2.268–70) describes pain in the ribs, and recommends the application of a metal or clay container filled with hot water, with something soft placed between container and skin to prevent further discomfort. It also discusses "dry fomentations", woollen envelopes filled with millet.

But what of the concept of pain underlying the use of painkillers? Is it possible to go behind the references to the kinds of substance used to relieve pain in the ancient world, and to say something about the specific medical, and general cultural, views of pain? First, specific medical attitudes to pain and pain relief. It is important to remember that ancient medicine was never one uniform system with a recognised training system, a fixed orthodoxy, and socially accepted qualifications. Instead, there were always many competing groups and individuals, sharing some ideas, but disagreeing on many areas[16, 17]. I have selected some texts from the Hippocratic corpus (5th to 3rd centuries BC) to illustrate the implications of some theoretical positions for the practice of pain relief.

A long discussion of pain (*odyne*) in a text called *Places in Man* (L 6.334–6) tells us that pain is produced by cold and hot, by excess and deficiency. It should at once be noted that the precise connotations of "hot" and "cold" are a little different from those in Dioscorides since, within the basic theme that life is "hot", this anonymous writer suggests that some people are naturally much hotter than others. In persons of a cold constitution pain is produced by heat, and in those of a hot constitution by cold. In the dry it is produced by wetness, in the wet by dryness. This is because pains are produced every time there is a change and corruption of the natural constitution (*physis*). Pains are therefore cured by contraries, each disorder (*nosema*) having a cure which is right for it. So hot constitutions, made sick by the cold, need a remedy which heats — and so on. This particular brand of ancient medicine, seeing everything in terms of the principle of opposites, would therefore not use any single substance as "a pain-killer", applicable to all situations; instead, the type of painkiller given would depend on the healer's assessment of the constitution of the patient.

Another text, *Epidemics* 6.6.3 (L 5.324), gives a series of general principles for relieving pain anywhere in the body; you should purge the nearest cavity of blood, using cautery or incision, or apply hot or cold substances, or induce sneezing, or use vegetable juices where these have power, or use the ancient multipurpose remedy called *kukeon*, a mixture of wine and flour. For even worse pains, milk, garlic, boiled wine, vinegar and salt are recommended. I would emphasise that the vegetable juices (*phyton chumoi*) are to be used "where these have power" — again implying that certain types of ancient medicine would regard as alien the idea of a drug having the same properties in all cases and situations.

Aphorisms 2.46 (L 4.48) says that if someone has two pains (*ponoi*), in different places, the stronger will cancel out the weaker; if this were to be applied to pain relief, it would suggest the principle that you create a worse pain somewhere else to remove the one you started with. Another text, *Diseases* 1.5 (L 6.148), suggests that doctors can relieve pain, but adds that pains often go away without any medical intervention; this text is generally concerned with the principle of chance in medicine, and also tells us that doctors may produce either a good or a disastrous outcome by chance alone.

There is thus no single medical attitude to the use of pain-relieving substances in antiquity. I would now like to turn to the general cultural context of pain and pain relief, concentrating on the ancient culture with which I am most familiar, that of classical Greece, the period of Hippocratic medicine.

There is an old idea that primitive peoples are less sensitive to pain; in fact the picture is far more complicated than this, since any culture will have certain situations in which the expression of pain is encouraged, and others in which stoicism is required[18]. Pain response may, thus, not be a fair reflection of the pain felt[19]. Pain accompanies normal physiological changes (e.g., childbirth) as well as injury and disease, and it can also be caused by the processes of diagnosis and healing themselves[20]. The ancient Greeks regarded pain as a central element in diagnosis, often giving its location as the first point in their lists of symptoms; thus for the Hippocratic writers, as for Galen, writing over 500 years later, pain was seen as an important indicator of the precise location of a disease[21]. They recognised that pain may be a natural part of some conditions and that sometimes the cessation of pain was far more dangerous than the pain itself: "Pains which go with no cause are fatal" (*KP* 19.364/L 5.660). They also acknowledged that the process of healing could cause pain; Plato implies that it is painful to take a drug and unpleasant to be treated by medicine, but adds that the pain must be endured if the patient is to recover (*Gorgias* 467c; 478b–c).

In my citation of the Hippocratic texts I have already drawn attention to two of the Greek words used for pain; *odyne* (as in our word "anodyne") and *ponoi*. Others include *algema/algos* (as in our word "analgesic") and *lype*. The extent to which one word for pain is used rather than another is partly a matter of the date and authorship of the treatise; thus, for example, *Epidemics* 7 and *Koan Prognoses* seem to prefer words of the *algos* group. Fabrega and Tyma, however, suggest a further class of factor governing the selection of word: cultural considerations, which mean that the words chosen can be used to tell us something of the idea of pain found in any particular culture. In English, "pain" derives from the Latin *poena*, "punishment"; thus, behind the word there is the idea of disease being caused by divine vengeance. The words used for pain will also act to shape the phenomenon of pain itself[22]. The fit between words and experiences may not be perfect; Diller's study[23] of Thai terms for pain reminds us that "lexical differentiation of pain terms might not correlate with physiological or psychological distinctions".

How can material such as this be applied to the ancient Greek texts? To an extent, in the medical texts *ponos* is often used for long-lasting pain, dull pain; *odyne* for sharp pain, pain which pierces the body. In this, *odyne* corresponds to the Thai term Diller classifies as PAIN$_3$, a "sudden piercing or stabbing pain, highly focused". To understand the field of meanings for *ponos* we must, however, look outside the medical texts. In classical studies there has been much work recently on the parallels drawn in ancient Greek culture between war, as the most highly-valued male social activity, and childbirth, as the activity by which women prove themselves to be proper women. According to Plutarch (*Life of Lycurgus* 27.2–3), the Spartans were allowed to commemorate only two classes of death by inscriptions on the tomb: men dying in battle, and women dying in childbirth. In a famous passage from Greek tragedy, Medea draws an explicit comparison between the two spheres of activity when she says that she would rather stand in the line of battle three times than give birth once (Euripides, *Medea* 248–51). This should probably not be taken as evidence that the Greeks expected normal childbirth to be more painful than battle injuries; Medea is not a typical Greek woman, but a foreign sorceress who murders her own children, and these lines occur in a long speech on the miserable condition of women, written by a man. However, both war and childbirth were seen as forms of combat involving pain, but in childbirth the enemy was labour itself[24]. Where this is the case — where some degree of pain is seen as a necessary part of the process — the idea of using any form of painkiller would perhaps be out of place[25]. The precise word used for pain in both war and childbirth is usually *ponos*, or the plural *ponoi*, but its use does not stop here.

One of the earliest uses of *ponos* is with the meaning "agricultural labour", "hard work". It is presented as an unpleasant, but integral, part of human existence, ordained by the gods and thus inescapable (e.g. Hesiod, *Works and Days* 92; 113). It hurts but, like war for men and childbirth for women, it is part of a process necessary for the continuation of human life. *Ponos* is also used for strengthening exercises — that is, for the training necessary for those who want to face the situations in which pain will occur. *Ponos* in its wider uses is thus pain with a goal, a means to an end, and I would suggest that this adds support to the suggestion that it is very unlikely to be relieved in any way. How can you relieve something divinely-ordained as part of the human condition? The parallels with the view from our own society's recent history, that childbirth must be painful because of Eve's role in the Fall from Eden, are clear.

59

If, however, we look closely at the early gynaecological and other medical texts, we discover something which may be significant. Labour pains are described not only as *ponoi*, but also as *odynai*. What do these alternatives signify? The text *Regimen in Acute Diseases* 7 (L 2.268–70) has already been discussed, but a further aspect of its description of fomentations for pain in the ribs is that, although it uses *odyne* for pain throughout, there is one exception to this pattern. This occurs when the writer warns, "but if warm fomentations do not relieve the *ponos*, do not continue using them, because they dry out the lung". Is *ponos* used here, too, with the sense "pain which cannot be relieved"? Such an analysis should not be pushed too far, since in some treatises there is a preference for *ponos* as the general word for "pain"; for example, in *Epidemics* 1.

The use of both terms for labour pains may then give us a hint — and I would emphasise that with these texts we cannot hope for more — that where childbirth was concerned there was some recognition that pain could be a necessary part of the process and thus had to be endured, but could also be excessive and thus required special attention. This is supported by *Diseases* 1.8 (L 6.154–6): a warning that, if a woman in labour has *odyne* in her womb and the doctor "gives her something" but she worsens or even dies, then he will be blamed. Drugs were then given to women in labour, in some cases, and it is interesting that it is *odyne* rather than *ponos* which is used here.

In our terms, some form of analgesia was administered to women whose pain was culturally defined as excessive. It was not only the doctor who would take the decision as to whether drugs should be given, since they were available to all members of ancient society, sold in the market place and at fairs[11]. Where pain relief was given by a doctor employed for the purpose, its efficacy would, however, have been improved by the whole ritual of consultation and therapy, as well as by the doctor's explanation of why it would work.

In conclusion, the example of labour pain suggests the limitations of any study of the early anodynes. In a culture which regarded much pain as a normal part of human life, patients may have been as reluctant to complain as healers were reluctant to administer painkilling drugs.

Acknowledgement

This work was completed during the tenure of a Sir James Knott Research Fellowship at the University of Newcastle.

References

1. Riddle, J. M. (1985). *Dioscorides on Pharmacy and Medicine*, p. xxii. Austin: University of Texas Press
2. Riddle, J. M. (1985). *Dioscorides on Pharmacy and Medicine*, pp 67–9. Austin: University of Texas Press
3. Shorter, E. (1983). *A History of Women's Bodies*, p. 187. London: Allen Lane
4. Lloyd, G. E. R. (1979). *Magic, Reason and Experience*, pp 46–7. Cambridge: Cambridge University Press
5. Hopkins, K. (1965). Contraception in the Roman Empire. *Comp. Stud. Soc. Hist.*, **8**, 124–51
6. Manuli, P. and Vegetti, M. (1977). *Cuore, Sangue e Cervello. Biologia e Antropologia nel Pensiero Antico*. Milan: Episteme
7. King, H. (1988). The daughter of Leonides: reading the Hippocratic corpus. In Cameron, A. (ed.) *History as Text*. London: Duckworth
8. Lloyd, G. E. R. (1983). *Science, Folklore and Ideology*, p. 83. Cambridge: Cambridge University Press
9. Riddle, J. M. (1985). *Dioscorides on Pharmacy and Medicine*, pp 107–8. Austin: University of Texas Press
10. Riddle, J. M. (1985). *Dioscorides on Pharmacy and Medicine*, p. 69. Austin: University of Texas Press
11. Nutton, V. (1985). The drug trade in antiquity. *J. Roy. Soc. Med.*, **78**, 138–45
12. Lloyd, G. E. R. (1983). *Science, Folklore and Ideology*, p. 128. Cambridge: Cambridge University Press
13. Nutton, V. (1985). The drug trade in antiquity. *J. Roy. Soc. Med.*, **78**, 142
14. Riddle, J. M. (1985). *Dioscorides on Pharmacy and Medicine*, pp 38 and 109. Austin: University of Texas Press
15. Lloyd, G. E. R. (1966). *Polarity and Analogy*, pp 44–5 and 62–3. Cambridge: Cambridge University Press

16. Lloyd, G. E. R. (1979). *Magic, Reason and Experience*, pp 89 ff. Cambridge: Cambridge University Press
17. Temkin, O. (1953). Greek medicine as science and craft. *Isis*, **44**, 213–25
18. Zborowski, M. (1952). Cultural components in responses to pain. *J. Soc. Issues*, **8**, 16–30
19. Wolff, B. B. and Langley, S. (1968). Cultural factors and the response to pain: a review. *Am. Anthropol.*, **70**, 494–501
20. Helman, C. (1984). *Culture, Health and Illness*, pp 95–105. Bristol: Wright
21. Siegel, R. E. (1970). *Galen on Sense Perception*, pp 184–93. Basel: Karger
22. Fabrega, H. F. and Tyma, S. (1976). Culture, language and the shaping of illness: an illustration based on pain. *J. Psychosomat. Res.*, **20**, 323–37
23. Diller, A. (1980). Cross-cultural pain semantics. *Pain*, **9**, 9–26
24. Loraux, N. (1975). Le lit, la guerre. *L'Homme*, **21**, 37–67
25. Zborowski, M. (1952). Cultural components in responses to pain. *J. Soc. Issues*, **8**, 18

Note: In this chapter the abbreviation "L" refers to the complete edition of the Hippocratic corpus edited by Emile Littré (10 volumes, Paris, 1839–1861; reprinted 1962, Amsterdam: Hakkert).

Chapter 4

The discovery and development of the contemporary anaesthetic agents

Patricia J. Flynn and James P. Payne

Before the advent of anaesthesia surgery was a ghastly and horrific business that almost certainly had a brutalising effect on most of those who practised it. Moreover, in almost every patient some degree of mutilation ensued and the case for surgery was not enhanced by the activities of the body-snatchers, such as Burke and Hare, who early in the 19th century provided the anatomy school in Edinburgh with corpses needed for dissection.

Whether one believes that the first anaesthetic in the UK was given in Dumfries or in London is scarcely relevant today. What is important is that almost immediately after the discovery of anaesthesia had been announced in the UK detailed accounts of its use were published. For example, within months of the announcement James Robinson[1], a London dentist, published his treatise on the inhalation of the vapour of ether for the prevention of pain in surgical operations.

Surgery was never to be the same again. The advent of anaesthesia allowed the surgeon to approach his task logically and methodically with time on his side. Nevertheless, even at the end of World War II the emphasis in anaesthesia was almost entirely on technical skill, with little or no consideration given to the scientific aspects of the subject. The anaesthetist's task was to provide an unconscious and motionless patient for the surgeon and he was not expected to concern himself

63

with any other aspect of the patient's welfare. However, with the growing complexity of modern surgical techniques and with the increasing tendency for surgeons to become engaged in heroic procedures, the anaesthetist has found himself in the role of the patient's protector against the surgical onslaught. If this appears a somewhat fanciful suggestion, it is worth reflecting on the fact that the fundamental distinction between the wound produced by the surgeon's scalpel and that inflicted by the mobster's knife is essentially one of motive; without the protection of anaesthesia the end result would be the same! Consider, for example, the patient who has his sternum split to allow access to his heart, which is then stopped to enable a congenital defect to be repaired or a diseased valve to be replaced. Without the protection afforded by the anaesthetist such a patient would have little chance of survival.

Today the anaesthetist is expected not only to render the patient unconscious but also to paralyse the respiratory muscles for the purpose of controlling respiration, to lower the blood pressure by the use of ganglion blocking drugs or some other technique in order to control bleeding, to reduce the body temperature as a protection against anoxia and even to arrest the circulation entirely. Once the operation has been successfully completed the anaesthetist then has the responsibility of supervising the postoperative management, with particular reference to pain relief, respiratory sufficiency and fluid replacement.

The purpose of this chapter is to focus on the advantages and disadvantages of the agents currently used in anaesthetic practice. Over the years nearly a score of inhalation agents have been used in clinical practice but up to the middle of the present century all had obvious disadvantages. Agents such as ether, ethyl chloride and cyclopropane were explosive, chloroform was hepatotoxic, trichloroethylene could cause nerve palsies if used inappropriately and most agents could produce cardiac dysrhythmias. Furthermore, for the most part a slow, troublesome and sometimes dangerous induction, a prolonged recovery and postoperative nausea and vomiting were accepted as inevitable components of a general anaesthetic which depended upon heavy dosage with a single agent.

The first breakthrough came when the use of an intravenous

induction with thiopentone[2] became standard practice; this was consolidated by the introduction of the natural alkaloid curare[3], to be followed by the synthetic neuromuscular blocking agents. Such a combination abolished the need for deep anaesthesia. The association of muscle relaxation with narcosis and analgesia provided what came to be known as balanced anaesthesia. Narcosis was obtained most commonly with intravenous thiopentone and analgesia with nitrous oxide supplemented by one or other of a range of inhalation agents or by pethidine. This triad of relaxation, narcosis and analgesia combined with controlled respiration soon became established as an effective means of maintaining anaesthesia for a wide range of surgical procedures. As with other methods, however, the technique was extended beyond its limit, with the result that some patients were able to describe parts of the operative procedure and even to repeat snatches of conversation between the operating room staff when interviewed after their return to the ward. Such a degree of awareness in a patient supposedly unconscious is difficult to justify and even if no harm is done, as has been claimed by some anaesthetists, because the analgesic action is still effective, there are better ways of providing analgesia if the patient wishes to remain awake.

The eclipse of the volatile agents such as ether, chloroform and cyclopropane by the nitrous oxide-oxygen-relaxant technique was suddenly reversed in 1956 when the introduction of the fluorinated hydrocarbon halothane[4] brought about the re-emergence of the classical inhalation method of anaesthesia[5]. Halothane, despite the criticism that it is responsible for severe liver damage in some patients, is still undoubtedly a most useful general purpose anaesthetic.

The effect of halothane on the liver is difficult to assess. When the original allegation that halothane was a liver poison became no longer tenable it was then claimed that in rare instances halothane could evoke a sensitivity-type hepatic reaction which was indistinguishable clinically, biochemically and histologically from ordinary acute viral hepatitis. Later it was asserted that such a distinction can be made but only if the pathologist is experienced!

It is perhaps significant that the term "halothane hepatitis" tends to be used not by anaesthetists but by specialists in internal medicine and pathologists whose experience and understanding of surgical and anaesthetic procedures leave much to be desired. It is equally significant that whereas the diagnosis of "halothane hepatitis" continues to be made by such specialists, often on the basis of ill-documented case reports and, on occasion, even in instances where the patient had not been exposed to halothane, extensive retrospective studies in Canada[6], in the UK[7] and in the USA[8] have failed to confirm the existence of such a disease entity. Even more significant, despite the millions of halothane anaesthetics administered, there is no single documented case of hepatitis following exposure to halothane alone that can be shown without reasonable doubt to be due to the drug.

There can be no question but that jaundice occasionally follows exposure to halothane, as it does after exposure to every other inhalational agent ever used. Those anaesthetists who were trained in the days before halothane will be familiar with the hepato-renal syndrome associated with ether anaesthesia. The argument therefore centres on whether postoperative hepatitis is a non-specific consequence of anaesthesia or whether it is a special effect of the administration of halothane. If such a reaction to halothane does occur, its incidence is so low as to be insignificant except on the rare occasions when a patient exposed to halothane develops postoperative malaise and fever that cannot be explained and then has to be anaesthetised again within a short time interval. In these circumstances the possibility that halothane can provoke a sensitivity-type reaction cannot be excluded. Unfortunately, however, the public utterances of individual physicians and some official bodies have tended to distort and magnify the problem so that anaesthetists are now being forced to make decisions based on medico-legal and political considerations rather than on their clinical judgement. Anaesthetists surely have a right to expect that if they cannot be helped by their colleagues in other disciplines at least their work should not be hampered by ill-informed comment, especially when matters of medico-legal importance are involved. Furthermore, if such specialists were to apply the same enthusiasm to the investigation of iatrogenic morbidity in their own fields of work, the gift of prophecy is not needed to forecast, for example, that the incidence of major problems after hepatic and renal biopsies would prove substantially higher than the incidence after halothane anaesthesia.

Halothane has been associated with another problem with a more general medical interest beyond anaesthesia. Malignant hyperpyrexia, a syndrome with a genetic origin and characterised by fever and usually by skeletal muscle rigidity triggered by the administration of suxamethonium or a potent inhalation agent such as halothane, has been described in recent years[9]. The relationship with halothane is almost certainly non-specific, since it has also been reported after ether and cyclopropane as well as after stress and exercise. With an incidence estimated at about 1 in 190 000 in the UK, it does not raise major difficulties, but with a mortality in excess of 60% those at risk need to be identified. It is more common in males than in females and in the young rather than in the old. The aetiology is unknown but clinical and experimental evidence indicates that the site of the defect is peripheral, and not central, and that the malignant hyperpyrexia is due to a genetic defect. A syndrome occurring in Landrace pigs is not only clinically identical with the human syndrome but also identical in many of the biochemical features.

At the time of its introduction, halothane was considered close to the ideal anaesthetic agent and it remains the ideal agent in certain clinical circumstances, notably paediatric airway problems. However, its known depression of respiratory and cardiovascular function encouraged further research for still better inhalation agents. That research came to be concentrated on the methyl-ethyl-ethers known to be associated with cardiac stability, and methoxyflurane was introduced in 1960. As predicted, it produced less cardiovascular depression than halothane and did not sensitise the myocardium to catecholamines. What was not predicted, however, was that biodegradation of methoxyflurane was much greater than that of halothane and the fluoride ion produced a dose-related toxic effect on renal function. Another fluorinated methyl-ethyl-ether, enflurane, was synthesised in 1963 and introduced into clinical practice in 1975. Enflurane's advantages over halothane include more rapid uptake and elimination, greater stability of cardiac rhythm and more profound muscle relaxation. Its disadvantages include relatively greater respiratory depression, abnormal electroencephalographic activity in certain circumstances and a degree of biodegradation to inorganic fluoride that may approach nephrotoxic levels in certain patients.

Isoflurane is the most recently introduced inhalational agent. It is an isomer of enflurane and was synthesised in 1965 but its introduction into clinical practice was delayed because of a potential risk of hepatic carcinogenicity which was not refuted until 1978[10]. The advantages of isoflurane over halothane include lower blood solubility and therefore more rapid recovery, stability of cardiac rhythm and minimal biodegradation. So far no evidence of serious toxicity has been detected, but since adverse effects have been reported for every volatile anaesthetic[11] it is surely only a matter of time before such reports appear.

Another area of concern about inhalational anaesthesia developed in the 1970s when a number of studies suggested an increased incidence of miscarriage and congenital abnormality in the offspring of staff exposed to waste anaesthetic gases, especially nitrous oxide. Most of these studies were retrospective, with questionable results with regard to accuracy of recall, reporter bias and difficulties in validation of information. A recent prospective study[12] of women doctors shows no relationship between specialty and incidence of abortion. It has been shown, however, that nitrous oxide inactivates vitamin B_{12} and may interfere with methionine synthetase and folate; it may thus produce megaloblastic bone marrow changes and agranulocytosis, in addition to neurological deficits. There is no evidence that these adverse effects occur in operating room staff, even when waste gases are not scavenged, or in surgical patients; however, the question arises as to whether nitrous oxide should be used in patients who are pregnant, severely infected or have poor wound healing. In addition, it has been suggested that nitrous oxide should not be used in patients given more than one anaesthetic at short intervals.

If the introduction of inhalation agents revolutionised surgery the impact of curare had a similar effect on anaesthetic practice. Those anaesthetists who began their training after the use of neuromuscular blocking drugs had become routine can have little understanding of the anaesthetic techniques used before that time. Until then a rapid smooth induction of anaesthesia and the maintenance of a steady state adequate for the surgical procedure was a work of art regularly accomplished by relatively few and then only after years of diligent practice[13]. This is no longer true. At best, unconsciousness can be achieved rapidly by the intravenous injection of a barbiturate or some other rapidly acting hypnotic and muscle relaxation can be induced immediately thereafter by the use of curare or a similar drug. At worst, the patient is at the mercy of any doctor, however unskilled, who can manage to put a needle into a vein.

On the subject of neuromuscular blocking drugs, Dr John Gillies[14], in his Joseph Clover Memorial Lecture, drew attention to the general improvement in anaesthetic practice brought about by their intro-duction. He went on to argue that with such drugs abolition of muscular tone was now easy and that, although certain difficulties and dangers still remained, conditions for the patient had improved and a considerable element of strain had been eliminated from the work of both the surgeon and the anaesthetist. These views were not universally accepted and in 1954 Beecher and Todd[15], in a somewhat sensational paper, alleged that the use of relaxants in the USA had increased anaesthetic deaths nearly 6-fold. In Europe, however, where large doses of curare were combined with nitrous oxide-oxygen anaesthesia and controlled ventilation, morbidity and mortality were substantially reduced, and it soon became obvious that the disparity was due to differences in technique. Early American practice did not take into account the need to artificially ventilate the lungs. Once this was corrected the American figures rapidly improved.

Among the difficulties and dangers that still persist one of the most obvious is the failure to reverse successfully the action of the curariform drugs by neostigmine. Respiratory depression and even respiratory arrest have been reported from time to time, particularly after neostigmine has been given in the recovery ward or in the intensive care unit, and this has been attributed to a so-called neo-stigmine-resistant curarisation. However, it is now clear that neostig-mine alone in doses commonly used clinically is capable of inducing neuromuscular block, with the implication that the neuromuscular block seen in such circumstances is not neostigmine-resistant but neostigmine-induced[16].

Despite the obvious advantages of curare it was not the ideal drug for clinical use. It is a naturally occurring compound and certainly in the initial stages standardisation was difficult. In addition, its lack of specificity produced side-effects such as hypotension and broncho-spasm, which occasionally led to problems in clinical management.

As a result chemists and pharmacologists began the search for more specific compounds free from the deficiencies of curare. Despite the quality of some of the new synthetic blocking drugs, the ideal compound has yet to be found. Nevertheless, within the past few years two new drugs, atracurium and vecuronium, have proved highly successful in clinical practice.

Atracurium was designed specifically to take advantage of a phenomenon well known to chemists, the Hofmann elimination mechanism, whereby the drug could be broken down at a pH and temperature within the physiological range and eliminated without the need to depend on either hepatic or renal pathways[17]. A particular advantage of atracurium is that its action is remarkably predictable and this, combined with the absence of cumulative effects, makes it very suitable for use as an infusion both in the operating room and in the intensive care unit[18].

Vecuronium[19,20], an analogue of pancuronium, a fairly long-acting neuromuscular blocking drug, has a duration and pattern of action comparable with atracurium. Like atracurium, it has also been used as an infusion in the operating room and in the intensive care unit. Vecuronium has one disadvantage: it is not stable in solution, so it is supplied in the dry state, to be dissolved immediately before use.

The problems of neuromuscular blockade are far from resolved but the amount of research currently in progress reflects the confidence of chemists and pharmacologists that new highly specific neuro-muscular blocking drugs, free from side-effects and tailored to meet the anaesthetist's requirements, will soon be available.

The recent emphasis on the use of infusions of neuromuscular blocking drugs is related to progress in the field of intravenous anaes-thesia, the history of which goes back to 1665 when Sir Christopher Wren described how he injected morphia into a ligated vein of a dog by means of a quill and a pig's bladder used as a syringe. The first serious attempts to develop intravenous anaesthesia were made during the period between the two World Wars after the introduction of a series of short-acting barbiturate drugs. Although hexobarbitone was the first to be used, and was an immediate success in 1932, it was overtaken two years later by thiopentone, which did not produce the involutionary muscle twitching seen with hexobarbitone. Despite the partial eclipse occasioned by the Pearl Harbour disaster[21], where the number of casualties who died was substantially increased by the indiscriminate use of barbiturate anaesthesia, thiopentone was soon re-established as the drug of choice for the induction of anaesthesia, a position it still holds today. It is perhaps surprising that thiopentone should have survived so long, since its properties are far from ideal, as witnessed by the extensive literature on the complications of intravenous anaesthesia. Nevertheless, among the barbiturates only methohexitone has achieved some popularity, mainly in outpatient anaesthesia and more controversially in dental practice.

The first non-barbiturate intravenous anaesthetic to be used clinically was propanidid, a eugenol derivative which showed promise, but because of problems of hypersensitivity related to the solubilising agent it has never become a serious rival to thiopentone. A similar fate befell althesin, a steroid anaesthetic which has now been withdrawn. For a time it seemed that etomidate might succeed where others had failed; introduced as a short-acting induction agent with a duration of effect of up to ten minutes, it has the disadvantage of having no analgesic action. Now that it has been shown to depress adrenocortical function when used as an infusion it seems unlikely to survive.

The present decade has seen the introduction for intravenous use of a relatively short-acting synthetic opiate, alfentanil[22], a similar short-acting benzodiazepine, midazolam[23], and a rapidly metabolised anaesthetic agent, propofol[24]. So far the only adverse reports have been related to a prolonged duration of action of alfentanil and midazolam and a slightly greater degree of respiratory and cardiovascular depression with propofol when compared with thiopentone. Propofol, an alkylphenol (2,6-diisoprohylphenol), is probably the most exciting anaesthetic drug to be made available in recent years and certainly promises to be the most effective challenge to the supremacy of thiopentone in the intravenous field. The onset of anaesthesia follows a pattern similar to that of thiopentone but the recovery process is quite distinctly different. Within 5–10 minutes after the termination of anaesthesia the patient is awake and responsive and within thirty minutes is fully alert and capable of reading a newspaper. Postoperative nausea and vomiting are very rare and, indeed, some patients volunteer the information that they are hungry and would enjoy a meal. The pattern after intravenous infusion is not significantly different and, unlike the case with thiopentone, there is no evidence of cumulative effects. It is perhaps too early yet to be dogmatic but experience to date suggests that propofol is set to change the pattern of anaesthetic practice, particularly in relation to day case surgery.

None of these advances would have been possible without the rapid expansion of technology in the post-war era. In particular, the design of calibrated vaporisers, the evolution of suitable stimulators for the assessment of neuromuscular block and the improvement in the quality of infusion pumps have all contributed to the present level of achievement. The development of anaesthetic technology has, however, brought its own problems, not the least of which are the steadily increasing costs and the dehumanising effect on medical care. On the question of cost it has been calculated that in most countries between one fifth and one tenth of the gross national product is spent on health care. In the UK about 6% of the nation's annual budget goes on the National Health Service, which reflects either the overall efficiency of the NHS or the parsimony of Government, or perhaps both. Undoubtedly, however, the most worrying aspect of the increase in technology is the decrease in contact between the clinician and the patient. As Ivan Illich[25] characteristically expressed it, "Until sickness came to be perceived as an organic or behavioural abnormality the patient could hope to find in the eyes of his doctor a reflection of his own anguish. What he now meets is the gaze of an accountant engaged in an input/output calculation. His sickness is taken from him and turned into the raw material for an institutional enterprise." It is not necessary to accept entirely Illich's interpretation of the situation to recognise the element of truth in his criticism. The fact that sympathetic understanding can often mean more to patients than superb technical achievement is not always appreciated by the specialist clinician, who may fail to recognise that what could be regarded logically as the trappings of care often mean more ɗo patients than the substance. For such patients the caring doctor is epitomised by Sir Luke Fildes' painting "The Doctor", which hangs in the Tate Gallery. The family doctor sitting anxiously at the bedside of the sick child is the public's image of what a good doctor should be and the profession ignores that at its peril.

72

It has to be accepted, however, that the much admired doctor-patient relationship is passing from the scene — if it was ever there! The increase in specialisation has meant that it is rare for any one doctor to have the complete care of the patient within his province. This is particularly true in anaesthesia, where there has been a tendency to concentrate on the technical achievements of the specialty rather than on the relief and comfort that the anaesthetist can provide for the patient whose fear of anaesthesia is probably greater than any other when he comes to be admitted to hospital. Quality of care demands attention to both aspects.

In terms of the doctor-patient relationship the anaesthetist is further disadvantaged in that he is seen for the most part as providing a service for another clinician. The result is that the patient is often unaware of the anaesthetist's contribution to the successful outcome of major surgery. Paradoxically perhaps, unlike most clinicians who merely prescribe drugs, anaesthetists are applied pharmacologists who not only personally administer extremely potent and potentially lethal substances but also remain with their patients until the effects have worn off. This may occur naturally by the processes of degradation and elimination or in some instances by the use of suitable antagonists to reverse, for example, the action of neuromuscular and ganglion blocking drugs. But whatever the means, the anaesthetist is there until the patient shows signs of recovering consciousness and his protective reflexes have returned.

In recent years there has been a tendency for anaesthetists to move out of the operating room to accept responsibility, for example, for the management of intensive care units and for the organisation of pain clinics. However, it needs to be remembered that the area of greatest risk is still the operating theatre and that has to remain the anaesthetist's primary responsibility.

References

1. Robinson, J. (1847). *A Treatise on the Inhalation of the Vapour of Ether for the Prevention of Pain in Surgical Operations*. London: Webster & Co.
2. Lundy, J. S. (1935). Intravenous anesthesia; preliminary report

of use of two new thiobarbiturates. *Proc. Staff Mtg, Mayo Clinic*, **10**, 536–43

3. Griffith, H. R. and Johnson, G. E. (1942). Use of curare in general anesthesia. *Anesthesiology*, **3**, 418–20
4. Raventos, J. (1956). The action of fluothane — a new volatile anaesthetic. *Br. J. Pharmacol.*, **11**, 394–410
5. Johnstone, M. (1956). The human cardiovascular response to fluothane anaesthesia. *Br. J. Anaesth.*, **28**, 392–410
6. Henderson, J. C. and Gordon, R. A. (1965). The incidence of postoperative jaundice with special reference to halothane. *Can. Anaesth. Soc. J.*, **11**, 453–9
7. Mushin, W. W., Rosen, M., Bowen, D. J. and Campbell, H. (1964). Halothane and liver dysfunction: a retrospective study. *Br. Med. J.*, **2**, 329–41
8. Summary of the National Halothane Study (1967). Possible association between halothane anesthesia and postoperative hepatic necrosis. *J. Am. Med. Assoc.*, **197**, 775–88
9. Britt, B. A. and Kalow, W. (1970). Malignant hyperthermia: aetiology unknown. *Can. Anaesth. Soc. J.*, **17**, 316–30
10. Eger 2nd, E. I., White, A. E., Brown, C. L., Biava, C. G., Corbett, T. H. and Stevens, W. C. (1978). A test of the carcinogenicity of enflurane, isoflurane, halothane, methoxyflurane and nitrous oxide in mice. *Anesth. Analg. (Cleve.)*, **57**, 678–94
11. Brown, B. R. and Gandolfi, A. J. (1987). Adverse effects of volatile anaesthetics. *Br. J. Anaesth.*, **59**, 14–23
12. Spence, A. A. (1987). Environmental pollution by inhalational agents. *Br. J. Anaesth.*, **59**, 96–103
13. Dripps, R. D. (1976). The clinician looks at neuromuscular blocking drugs. In Zaimis, E. (ed.) *Neuromuscular Junction*, pp 583–92. Berlin, Heidelberg and New York: Springer-Verlag
14. Gillies, J. (1950). Anaesthetic factors in the causation and prevention of excessive bleeding during surgical operations. *Ann. Roy. Coll. Surg. Engl.*, **7**, 204–21
15. Beecher, H. K. and Todd, D. P. (1954). A study of the deaths associated with anesthesia and surgery. *Ann. Surg.*, **140**, 2–34
16. Payne, J. P., Hughes, R. and Al Azawi, S. (1980). Neuromuscular blockade by neostigmine in anaesthetized man. *Br. J. Anaesth.*,

52, 69–76

17. Stenlake, J. B., Waigh, R. D., Urwin, J., Dewar, G. H. and Coker, G. G. (1983). Atracurium: conception and inception. *Br. J. Anaesth.*, **55**, 3–10S

18. Payne, J. P. and Hughes, R. (1981). Evaluation of atracurium in anaesthetised man. *Br. J. Anaesth.*, **53**, 45–54

19. Savage, D. S., Sleigh, T. and Carlyle, I. (1980). The emergence of ORG NC 45, 1-(2α, 3α, 5α, 16β, 17β)-3-17 bis(acetyloxy)-2-(1-piperidinyl)-androstan-16-yl)-1-methyl piperidinium bromide, from the pancuronium series. *Br. J. Anaesth.*, **52**, 3–9S

20. Crul, J., and Booij, L. D. H. J. (1980). First clinical experiences with ORG NC 45, *Br. J. Anaesth.*, **52**, 49S

21. Halford, F. J. (1943). A critique of intravenous anesthesia in war surgery. *Anesthesiology*, **4**, 67–9

22. Kay, B. (1983). Alfentanil. In Bullingham, R. E. S. (ed.) *Clinics in Anesthesiology*, No. 1, pp 143–6. London, Philadelphia and Toronto: W. B. Saunders

23. Dundee, J. W., Halliday, N. J., Harper, K. W. and Brogden, R. N. (1984). Midazolam, a review of its pharmacological properties and therapeutic use. *Drugs*, **28**, 519–43

24. Editorial (1985). Propofol ('Diprivan'): A new intravenous anaesthetic. In Healy, T. E. J., Hoffbrand, B. I., Kay, B., Oakes, A. E. M., McAinsh, J., Glen, J. B. and Stark, R. D. (eds) *Postgrad. Med. J.*, **61**, Suppl. 3

25. Illich, I. (1975). *Medical Nemesis. The Expropriation of Health.* London: Marion Boyard Publishers Ltd

Chapter 5

The history of the non-steroidal anti-inflammatory agents

R. D. Mann

The drugs which began today's non-steroidal anti-inflammatory agents (NSAIDs) were botanical substances used in antiquity. The modern history of this group of drugs, which is now vastly used for the relief of pain, commenced about a hundred years ago when the synthesised drugs phenazone, amidopyrine and acetylsalicylic acid entered clinical practice. The experience of today's NSAIDs spans the last twenty-five years or so, during which many of these drugs have entered therapeutics and data on the adverse reactions associated with their use have been accumulated.

The origins of phenylbutazone

The search that ultimately produced phenylbutazone and a number of fairly closely related drugs began with 19th century efforts to find substitutes for quinine. Quinine had become widely popular in the treatment of fevers and its price had risen with the reduction of supply resulting from the uncontrolled cutting of the Peruvian cinchona trees. It was then found that the molecule of quinine contained benzene rings, and quinoline was isolated. The fascinating story of the discovery and early use of quinine has been told elsewhere[1]. It is perhaps most enjoyably read in the little work called *A Memoir of the*

Lady Ana de Osorio, Countess of Chinchon and Vice-Queen of Peru (AD 1629–39) ... which was published by Clements R. Markham[2] in 1874.

The 19th century search for antipyretics and analgesics also led to the examination of substances derived from coal tar. The preparation of carbolic acid, or phenol, was first reported in 1834 by Friedlieb Ferdinand Runge (1795–1867)[3]. Its antiseptic properties were described in 1860 by François Jules Lemaire (1814–1886)[4]. Lemaire had, in fact, noted that phenol was a powerful disinfectant and he entitled his study "Du coaltar saponiné, désinfectant énergique". Joseph Lister (1827–1912)[5,6], once he had fully realised the significance of the discoveries of Louis Pasteur (1822–1895) regarding fermentation, used phenol in introducing the antiseptic principle into surgery. In the *Lancet* of 1867 he published his essay "On a new method of treating compound fracture, abscess, ... "; later, again in 1867 and in the *Lancet*, he printed his epoch-making paper "On the antiseptic principle in the practice of surgery". In addition to its antiseptic action, phenol was thought, as a result of accidental observations, to be capable of lessening fever.

In this respect it resembled aniline, which was isolated from coal tar by William Henry Perkin (1838–1907), thus beginning the great aniline dye industry. It was soon appreciated that both phenol and aniline were far too toxic to be used systemically. Attempts to lessen the toxicity of aniline (phenylamine; aminobenzene) and phenol (hydroxybenzene) produced the fertile observation that the toxicity of these substances (and of salicylic acid) was lessened by simple acetylation.

The search for substitutes for quinine continued. Early attempts involved the synthesis of a variety of tetrahydroquinoline compounds, some of which were, for a short time, used clinically. Then, in the spring of 1875, while working in Strasburg, Emil Fischer (1852–1919) — when still only 23 years old — unintentionally synthesised the novel chemical substance, phenylhydrazine. Fischer, born in Rhenish Prussia, became successively professor of chemistry at Munich (1879), Erlangen (1882), Würzburg (1885) and Berlin (1892). In Munich he undertook a celebrated set of researches into the reactions of phenylhydrazine. These brilliant studies permitted the synthesis of a whole series of cyclic compounds with nitrogen atoms incorporated in the ring structures.

Fischer continued these experiments in early heterocyclic chemistry after his move to Erlangen. One of his assistants, Ludwig Knorr (1859–1921), by reacting phenylhydrazine with acetoacetic acid, produced a compound which he (wrongly) thought to be a tetra-hydroquinoline. After discussion with Wilhelm Filehne (1844–1927), who at that time had an interest in tetrahydroquinolines used as anti-pyretics, he produced the N-methylated derivative of his original compound. This was found to be less irritant than either quinine or salicylic acid. Knorr gave the patent rights to the Hoechst dye works and his compound entered clinical use under the trade name "Anti-pyrine".

In 1884 Knorr[7] showed that Antipyrine (phenazone; dimethyl phenyl pyrazoline) was, in fact, a pyrazoline derivative. After its introduction into clinical use by Filehne[8] in 1884, the drug swept Europe, becoming widely used, until it was slowly replaced by acetylsalicylic acid. Antipyrine was to no small extent responsible for the massive 19th century growth of some segments of the German pharmaceutical industry.

Filehne[9], attempting to improve on the antipyretic agents developed in his laboratory, went on to produce the dimethyl amino derivative of Antipyrine and in 1896 he introduced the newly synthesised amido-pyrine (aminophenazone) under the trade name "Pyramidon". Both Antipyrine and Pyramidon (Figure 1) were early noted to have anti-inflammatory as well as antipyretic activity. Regrettably, prior to World War II both were suspected of causing fatal agranulocytosis and other blood dyscrasias.

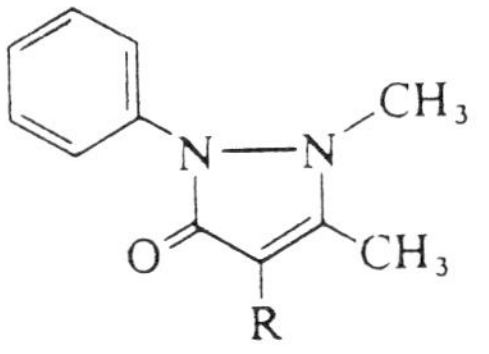

Phenazone,   R = −H
Amidopyrine, R = −N(CH₃)₂

Figure 1   Chemical structure of phenazone and amidopyrine

In 1952 a 4-butyl, 2-phenyl derivative of Antipyrine, phenylbuta-zone[10], was introduced into clinical medicine by the Swiss pharma-ceutical company, J. R. Geigy A. G. Phenylbutazone was given the trade name "Butazolidin"; it was of undoubted and singular efficacy and achieved enormous world-wide usage. The adverse experience associated with its use will be discussed later. It is enough for present purposes to note that Martindale[11], in discussing amidopyrine, states: "... the risk of agranulocytosis in patients taking amidopyrine is sufficiently great to render this drug unsuitable for use. Onset of agranulocytosis may be sudden and unpredictable." In respect of phenylbutazone, the same source[12] records that the "more severe reactions include reactivation of gastric and duodenal ulcers with perforation, haematemesis and melaena, hepatitis, hypertension, and, more rarely, agranulocytosis, thrombocytopenia, and aplastic anaemia."

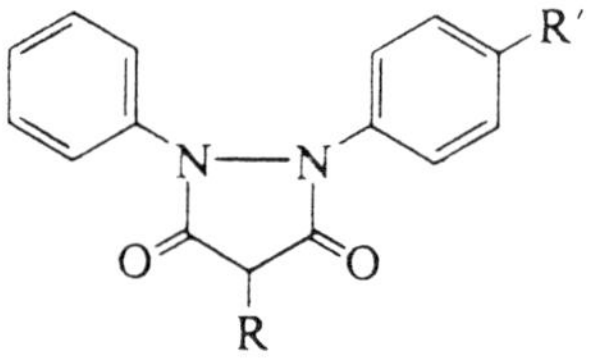

	R	R'
Phenylbutazone	$-CH_2CH_2CH_2CH_3$	$-H$
Oxyphenbutazone	$-CH_2CH_2CH_2CH_3$	$-OH$
Feprazone	$-CH_2CH=C(CH_3)_2$	$-H$

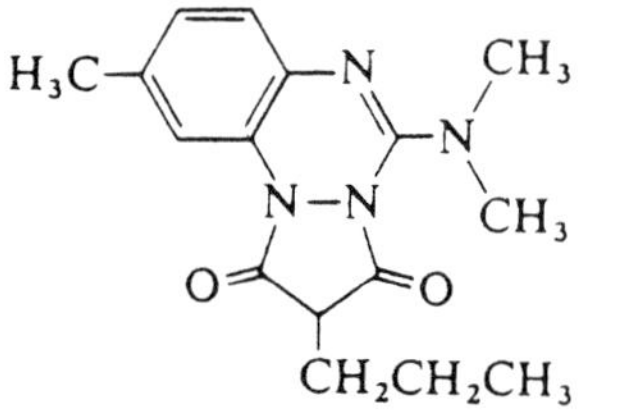

Azapropazone

Figure 2   Structure of phenylbutazone and related compounds, and of azapropazone

Two compounds which are chemically related to phenylbutazone have since been marketed; these are (Figure 2) azapropazone (apazone; "Rheumox") and feprazone ("Methrazone"). The active metabolite of phenylbutazone, oxyphenbutazone ("Tanderil"), was also marketed in the late 1950s. It offered no advantage over phenylbutazone and in 1984 was withdrawn from clinical use at the time when, due to its adverse reactions profile, phenylbutazone was restricted to use in hospitals for the treatment of ankylosing spondylitis. Feprazone has also been withdrawn from clinical use.

The story of the lineage of phenylbutazone is an example of the commonplace observation that the search for new, patentable drugs often begins with substances of known modest activity and acceptable toleration and then, by adjustments to the molecular structure, attempts to produce substances of improved activity and/or lessened toxicity. In the case of phenylbutazone it can be doubted if the story of such attempts has been a happy one.

The development of acetylsalicylic acid

The willow (Figure 3) was noted in antiquity. The Old Testament book of Leviticus[13] speaks of the "willows of the brook …" and Willow Bark, the bark of *Salix alba* and other species, notably *Salix fragilis*, of the Salicaceae, was still a monographed item in the *British Pharmaceutical Codex*[14] of 1934. It has been said[15] that in ancient times "the willow leaves or bark were crushed in olive oil and applied from specially formed clay pots to painful joints".

It has been widely acknowledged that the first, in modern times, to call attention to the beneficial properties of the willow was the Reverend Edmund Stone[16], whose publication in the *Philosophical Transactions of the Royal Society* in 1763 is reproduced in Appendix 1. Edmund Stone, attracted by the Doctrine of Signatures ("that many natural maladies carry their cures along with them"), found the willow to be "very efficacious in curing aguish and intermitting disorders". His experience was probably of malaria and other intermittent fevers and he tested the willow in some fifty patients after recording that its "extraordinary bitterness" made him think of the Peruvian bark, the source of quinine.

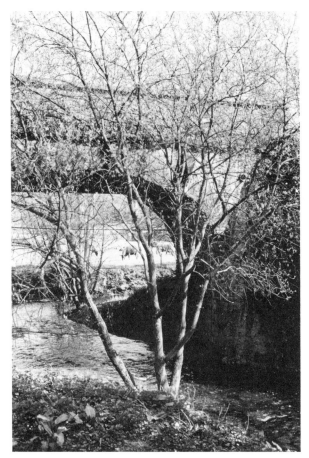

Figure 3   The willow, *Salix alba*

Willow bark achieved practical use. Samuel Jones[17], a surgeon of Hoddesdon, Hertfordshire, in 1792 reported the "singular efficacy in the cure of agues" of a particular species of willow. In 1798 Mr William White[18], an apothecary in Bath, reported being able to save at least £20 for the charity by substituting willow bark for Peruvian bark. He recorded the use of the willow in twenty-four cases and mentioned rheumatism in the last one of these only. He thought "the good effects of the willow seem entirely to arise from its tonic property, whilst those of the cinchona are owing to a peculiar modification of tonic and antiseptic qualities". About the same time, in 1803, G. Wilkinson[19] of Sunderland endorsed the efficacy of the willow.

These authors had all used willow bark as an antipyretic, at the time when acute rheumatic illnesses were still being treated with purgatives and by repeated venesection.

The active principle of willow bark is the glycoside, salicin, which itself retained a place in the *British Pharmameuctical Codex*[20] of 1934. H. Leroux[21] found salicin in willow bark in 1830. The substance was isolated by Raffaele Piria (1815–1865)[22] and in 1839 Piria reported the preparation of salicylic acid (*ortho*-hydroxybenzoic acid) from salicin. Salicylic acid was then synthesised by H. Gerland[23] in 1852. It was introduced into clinical use as an antipyretic in 1875, by Carl Emil Buss[24], who, at St Gallen in Switzerland, administered it to typhoid patients as an internal disinfectant. His careful and detailed observations showed an antipyretic effect despite the fact that the drug did not cure the typhoid infection.

It was left to Thomas J. Maclagan[25, 26] of Dundee to report in 1876 the specific usefulness of salicin in acute rheumatism. Maclagan, like the Reverend Edmund Stone before him, was attracted by the Doctrine of Signatures. He wrote:

"It seemed to me that a remedy for that disease would most hopefully be looked for among those plants and trees whose favourite habitat presented conditions analogous to those under which the rheumatic miasm seemed most to prevail. A low-lying, damp locality, with a cold, rather than warm, climate, give(s) the conditions under which rheumatic fever is most readily produced. On reflection, it seemed to me that the plants whose haunts best correspond to such a description were those belonging to the natural order Salicaceae, the various forms of willow. Among the Salicaceae, therefore, I determined to search for a remedy for acute rheumatism. The bark of many species of willow contains a bitter principle called salicin. This principle was exactly what I wanted."

In the same year (1876) Solomon Stricker (1834–1898)[27] of Berlin noted that sodium salicylate appeared to be able to arrest acute rheumatic fever. Striker published his results on 21st February 1876, shortly before Maclagan's first paper on salicin appeared in the *Lancet*. Maclagan, whose paper[25] was dated 4th March 1876, recorded that "the idea of treating acute rheumatism by salicin occurred to me in November 1874".

By this time, acetylsalicylic acid (*ortho*-acetoxybenzoic acid) was already known. It had first been produced in 1853 by Charles Gerhardt (1816–1856)[28], Professor of Chemistry at Strasburg. Strangely, this event — the synthesis of today's most widely used drug — aroused no initial interest. It is perhaps curious to reflect that acetylsalicylic acid had already been known to the literature for twenty-three years before the usefulness of the salicylates in acute rheumatism was clearly described.

The eventual introduction of acetylsalicylic acid into medical practice has been frequently described but remains of unusual interest. It is said that Heinrich Dreser (1860–1925)[29], Director of Research of Friedrich Bayer & Co. at Elberfeld, and previously Professor of Chemistry at Göttingen, wished to find for use by a relative or associate a form of salicylate which would be less irritating to the stomach than the sodium salicylate then available. One of the Bayer chemists, Felix Hoffman, is credited[30,31] with having undertaken a literature search on the salicylates — and this revealed acetylsalicylic acid. Dreser then demonstrated the relative lack of local irritation from acetylsalicylic acid by using the gills of live goldfish — a fairly early example of animal safety evaluation. Bayer selected "Aspirin" as the trade name for acetylsalicylic acid and the substance was introduced into clinical medicine in 1899. The chemical formula, compared with that of salicin, is shown in Figure 4.

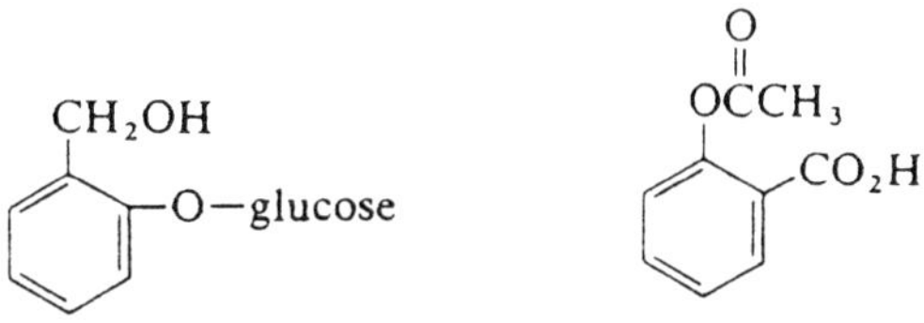

Figure 4 Chemical structure of salicin and aspirin

During World War I the British Government offered a reward for the development of a workable manufacturing process, even if this infringed the still valid Bayer patent for acetylsalicylic acid, which was then no longer available from Germany. American chemists could not compete as their country was not at war with Germany. The eventual result was the process by which George Nicholas, a pharmacist of Melbourne, brought in the "Aspro" tablets which, after the war, competed with the Bayer "Aspirin" product. After legal actions and post-war events of sequestration, Bayer lost the exclusive use of the trade-mark "Aspirin", and this term subsequently became the approved name for the product in the *British Pharmacopoeia*.

The newer non-steroidal anti-inflammatory agents

There has always been clinical concern regarding the degree of gastric irritation associated with the use of acetylsalicylic acid in the large doses needed to control severe rheumatic conditions. This, and the toxicity of the steroid hormones themselves, associated with the massive size of the market for analgesics and antipyretics, provided an incentive for further pharmaceutical development.

The first of the alternatives to acetylsalicylic acid was mefenamic acid ("Ponstan")[32], which has a remote chemical relationship to salicylic acid. The drug (Figure 5), developed by Parke, Davis & Co., is still in use. The chemically-related flufenamic acid ("Meralen") has been withdrawn from use, unlike the related drug, diclofenac ("Voltarol"), which remains available.

The idea that the indolic hormone, serotonin (5-hydroxytrypt-amine), might be involved in the inflammatory process led to the

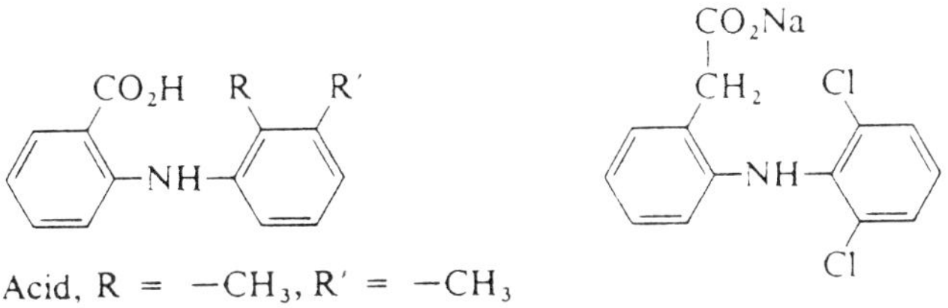

Mefenamic Acid, R = $-CH_3$, R′ = $-CH_3$
Flufenamic Acid, R = $-H$, R′ = $-CF_3$

Diclofenac

Figure 5 Chemical structure of mefenamic acid, flufenamic acid and diclofenac

85

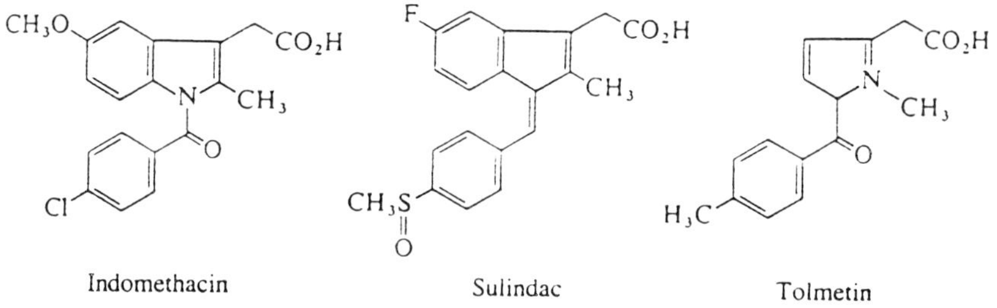

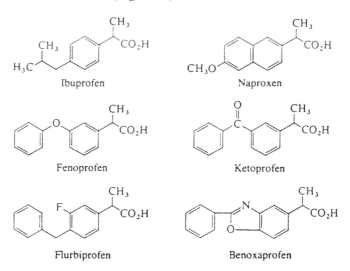

Figure 6   Chemical structure of indomethacin, sulindac and tolmetin

screening in animals of large numbers of indole compounds. The best of those examined at the Merck Institute at West Point, Pennsylvania, was introduced in 1963 as indomethacin ("Indocid")[33]. Attempts to find better tolerated chemical relatives led to the introduction (Figure 6) of sulindac ("Clinoral") and tolmetin ("Tolectin").

The view that a carboxylic acid group might play an important part in the useful activity of acetylsalicylic acid led to the screening by chemists of the Boots Pharmaceutical Company of a number of carboxylic acid derivatives, many of which were already available. The eventual outcome (Figure 7) was the introduction in 1964 of

Figure 7   Chemical structure of ibuprofen and various later phenylpropionic acid derivatives

ibuprofen ("Brufen")[34]. Later phenylpropionic acid derivatives have included fenoprofen ("Fenopron"), ketoprofen ("Orudis"; "Alrheumat"), naproxen ("Naprosyn"), flurbiprofen ("Froben") and benoxaprofen ("Opren"). The vastly different adverse reaction reporting experience with this range of drugs is reviewed later. Benoxaprofen was withdrawn following recognition of its adverse effects profile.

Other introductions (Figure 8) have included salicylate derivatives, benorylate ("Benoral") and diflunisal ("Dolobid"), and the oxicams, of which the most notable has been piroxicam ("Feldene")[35]. Piroxicam has been associated with many reports of serious gastrointestinal haemorrhage of which it has been the suspect cause. The drug is the first clinically useful member of the anti-inflammatory benzothiazine carboxamides (the oxicams). Some members of the compounds studied in the Pfizer programme which eventually produced piroxicam had marked effects on prothrombin time[35]. It is perhaps important that the published clinical literature is imprecise regarding any such clinical effects in elderly patients given piroxicam.

The early history of the anti-rheumatic drugs has been reviewed by Rodnan and Benedek (1970)[36]. More recently, an excellent account of the development of these drugs has been given by Walter Sneader (1985)[30] of the University of Strathclyde. Rainsford (1985)[37] has edited an extensive 3-volume study of the modern anti-inflammatory and anti-rheumatic drugs.

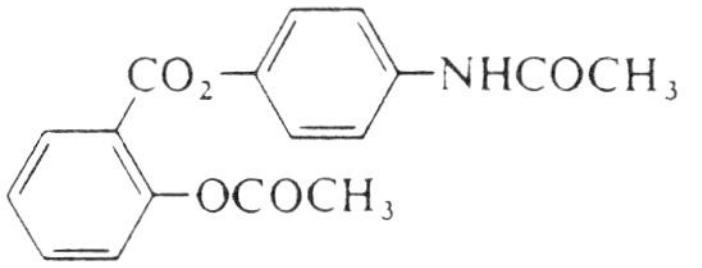

Benorylate

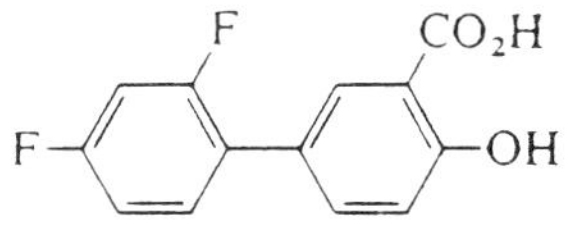

Diflunisal

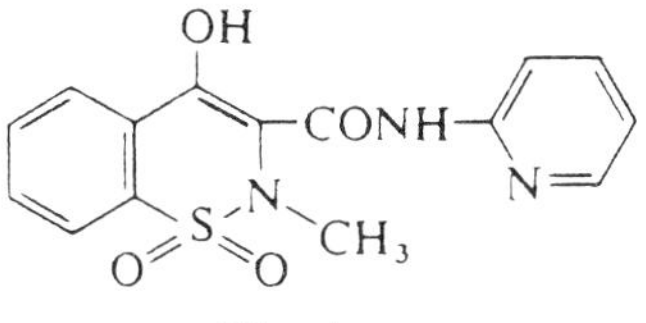

Piroxicam

Figure 8   Chemical structure of benorylate, diflunisal and piroxicam

The adverse reactions experience with the NSAIDs in the UK

The Committee on Safety of Medicines (CSM) maintains an Adverse Reactions Register in order to fulfil its statutory obligations under the Medicines Act, 1968. This Register was begun in 1964 by the Committee on Safety of Drugs (the Dunlop Committee), the fore-runner of the CSM. The data are collected principally by means of the yellow card notification scheme which has recently been extensively reviewed elsewhere[38]. The yellow cards are completed by doctors and dentists who wish to report suspected adverse reactions. They are collected centrally and the data are carefully assessed, collated and analysed.

Reports on suspected reactions with the NSAIDs have always been numerous. To take one example: in men the NSAIDs were the suspected cause in 233 (24.7%) of the 944 *serious* reactions reported in 1985; in women these drugs were the suspected cause in 433 (29.8%) of the 1455 *serious* reactions notified in the same year. The most important of the serious suspected reactions involving the NSAIDs are now gastrointestinal bleeding and perforation. Between 1964 and 1985 the Committee on Safety of Medicines received approximately 3500 reports of upper gastrointestinal bleeding or perforation sus-pected of being caused by these drugs. Over 600 of these reports involved deaths and about 90% of these fatal events were in patients aged 60 years or older. These disturbing figures indicate the scale of the relevant problem. Such problems are difficult to deal with as, in the absence of case–control studies of adequate size and appropriate design, the data from spontaneous adverse drug reaction reporting systems are difficult to interpret if the presenting clinical condition thought to be drug-related is, in any case, spontaneously fairly common in patients of the relevant age group.

In 1986 the Committee on Safety of Medicines published figures showing the number of reports (and deaths) of serious gastrointestinal suspected reactions and other (liver, kidney, skin and blood) serious suspected reactions in which the different NSAIDs were involved. These data, covering the period 1964 to 1985 and amounting to a total of 6097 reports of serious reactions, including 1247 deaths, are reproduced in Table 1.

Table 1 Number of reports (and deaths) of serious gastrointestinal suspected reactions, haemorrhage and perforation, and other serious suspected reactions of the liver, kidney, skin and blood. (Reproduced, with permission, from *Br. Med. J.*, 1986, **292**, 1190)

Drug (year marketed)	Serious gastrointestinal reactions	Other serious reactions	Total serious reactions
Aspirin (1899)	192 (71)	26 (7)	218 (78)
Phenylbutazone (1952)	222 (71)	688 (326)	910 (397)
Mefenamic acid (1963)	26 (1)	167 (21)	193 (22)
Indomethacin (1964)★	324 (126)	226 (48)	550 (174)
Oxyphenbutazone (1965)	13 (3)	241 (116)	254 (119)
Ibuprofen (1969)	218 (29)	163 (15)	381 (44)
Alclofenac (1972)	2 (0)	15 (2)	17 (2)
Naproxen (1973)	336 (40)	138 (21)	474 (61)
Ketoprofen (1973)	225 (17)	42 (3)	267 (20)
Fenoprofen (1974)	82 (9)	56 (11)	138 (20)
Azapropazone (1976)	150 (22)	64 (3)	214 (25)
Sulindac (1977)	37 (7)	62 (2)	99 (9)
Flurbiprofen (1977)	140 (15)	43 (5)	183 (20)
Feprazone (1978)	23 (0)	61 (5)	84 (5)
Diflunisal (1978)	122 (11)	49 (3)	171 (14)
Fenclofenac (1978)	23 (4)	61 (5)	84 (9)
Diclofenac (1979)	126 (17)	99 (2)	225 (19)
Tolmetin (1979)	4 (0)	4 (0)	8 (0)
Fenbufen (1980)	72 (4)	74 (7)	146 (11)
Piroxicam (1980)	641 (62)	121 (12)	762 (74)
Benoxaprofen (1980)	113 (19)	219 (58)	332 (77)
Zomepirac (1981)	68 (3)	20 (4)	88 (7)
Tiaprofenic Acid (1982)	55 (6)	6 (0)	61 (6)
Indoprofen (1982)	50 (7)	0 (0)	50 (7)
"Osmosin" (1982)	170 (26)	8 (0)	178 (26)
Suprofen (1983)	9 (1)	1 (0)	10 (1)

★Excluding Osmosin brand of indomethacin

These crude totals need to be related to some measure or other of drug use and to some standard period of marketing experience. The latter must allow for the fact that doctors are asked to report all reactions with new drugs but serious reactions only with older drugs. Table 2 relates the number of reports of serious suspected reactions to the prescription volume — both factors being considered over the first five years of marketing of each drug shown. The table needs to be

Table 2 Prescription-related reports (and deaths) of serious suspected gastrointestinal and other serious suspected reactions of the liver, kidney, skin and blood to some non-steroidal anti-inflammatory agents during their first five years of marketing. (Reproduced, with permission, from *Br. Med. J.*, 1986, **292**, 1191)

Drug	No. of serious gastrointestinal reactions	No. of other serious reactions	Prescriptions (million)	Gastrointestinal reactions per million prescriptions	Other serious reactions per million prescriptions	Total serious reactions per million prescriptions
Benoxaprofen*	113 (19)	219 (58)	1.47	76.9 (12.9)	149.0 (39.5)	225.9 (52.4)
Fenclofenac	20 (3)	50 (3)	0.53	37.7 (5.7)	94.3 (5.7)	132.1 (11.3)
Feprazone	22 (0)	56 (5)	0.44	50.0 (0)	127.3 (11.4)	177.3 (11.4)
Indoprofen*	50 (7)	0 (0)	0.09	555.6 (77.8)	0 (0)	555.6 (77.8)
"Osmosin"*	170 (26)	8 (0)	0.44	386.4 (59.1)	18.2 (0)	404.5 (59.1)
Azapropazone	61 (7)	19 (2)	0.91	67.0 (7.7)	20.9 (2.2)	87.9 (9.9)
Diclofenac	68 (9)	60 (1)	3.25	20.9 (2.8)	18.5 (0.3)	39.4 (3.1)
Diflunisal	105 (8)	43 (3)	3.13	33.5 (2.6)	13.7 (1.0)	47.2 (3.5)
Fenbufen†	56 (3)	53 (4)	1.57	35.7 (1.9)	33.8 (2.5)	69.4 (4.5)
Fenoprofen	54 (7)	19 (4)	1.67	32.3 (4.2)	11.4 (2.4)	43.7 (6.6)
Flurbiprofen	92 (7)	28 (4)	3.35	27.4 (2.1)	8.4 (1.2)	35.8 (3.3)
Ketoprofen	106 (5)	17 (0)	3.19	33.2 (1.6)	5.3 (0)	38.6 (1.6)
Naproxen	153 (19)	39 (7)	4.67	32.8 (4.1)	8.4 (1.5)	41.1 (5.6)
Piroxicam	538 (48)	86 (9)	9.16	58.7 (5.2)	9.4 (1.0)	68.1 (6.2)
Sulindac	33 (5)	42 (2)	1.38	23.9 (3.6)	30.4 (1.4)	54.3 (5.1)
Suprofen*	8 (1)	1 (0)	0.05	160.0 (20.0)	20.0 (0)	180.0 (20.0)
Tiaprofenic Acid*	45 (6)	3 (0)	0.60	75.0 (10.0)	5.0 (0)	80.0 (10.0)
Tolmetin	5 (0)	3 (0)	0.12	41.7 (0)	25.0 (0)	66.7 (0)
Ibuprofen	36 (3)	36 (1)	5.47	6.6 (0.5)	6.6 (0.2)	13.2 (0.7)

*Marketed for less than five years

†See editor's note on page 119.

considered with care, for reports seldom prove causation in individual patients and the drugs were marketed at very different periods during the twenty-three years covered by the yellow card scheme. Drugs for which prescription data are not available from the Prescription Pricing Authority for the first five years of marketing have been omitted from Table 2. Incomplete reporting, the fact that some of these drugs had less than five years of marketing history, the fact that the number of prescriptions greatly exceeds the number of patients due to repeat prescribing, and the fact that serious gastrointestinal adverse events occur fairly frequently in the late years of life even in the absence of drug therapy, all need to be kept in mind in examining Table 2.

Taking into account all these potential confounding factors, the Committee on Safety of Medicines[39] felt that the following three broad conclusions could be drawn from the data then available:

"As a group non-steroidal anti-inflammatory drugs are an important cause of serious adverse reactions.

The adverse reaction profile of individual drugs varies. Some cause predominantly gastrointestinal reactions, while others have a greater effect on the blood, liver, kidney, or skin.

The toxicity of marketed non-steroidal anti-inflammatory drugs varies between products, and the CSM considers that these drugs fall into three categories. Five products (benoxaprofen, fenclofenac, feprazone, indoprofen, and Osmosin (slow release indomethacin)) appeared to be substantially more toxic than others and have been withdrawn. One product (ibuprofen) appears to be less toxic, at least at low dosage, and is now available from pharmacies without prescription. In terms of overall safety the remaining drugs cannot be clearly distinguished from each other on the basis of yellow card reports. It is not yet possible to determine whether the apparent differences between these drugs are due to their toxicity or to confounding factors and reporting bias. Comparisons with suprofen are especially difficult because it is the newest of the drugs and postmarketing experience in Britain is therefore limited."

Suprofen has been withdrawn since these conclusions were published[39] and since, in May 1986, the Committee gave the following advice:

"Non-steroidal anti-inflammatory drugs should not be given to patients with active peptic ulceration.

In patients with a history of peptic ulcer disease and in the elderly they should be given only after other forms of treatment have been carefully considered.

In all patients it is prudent to start at the bottom end of the dose range."

The data given in Tables 1 and 2 can be seen in context by taking the overall data for 1985 as an example. In that year, as shown in Table 3, the NSAIDs accounted for 666 (27.8%) of the 2399 serious suspected reactions which were reported and these 2399 serious reactions comprised 19.1% of the total 12 541 suspected reactions of all grades of severity reported with all drugs in Britain.

The totals for serious reactions associated with NSAIDs in 1985 are actually a little lower than for the immediately preceding years, as can be appreciated from Figure 9. This figure also demonstrates that in each of the years since 1964, when the yellow card reporting scheme began, the number of serious reports related to this group of drugs has been greater in women than in men. The great increase in the

Table 3 Total number of yellow card reports, 1985

	All drugs, all reactions	All drugs, serious reactions	NSAIDs, serious reactions
Males	4 545	944	233
Females	7 996	1 455	433
Total	12 541	2 399	666
	– 19.1% –	– 27.8% –	

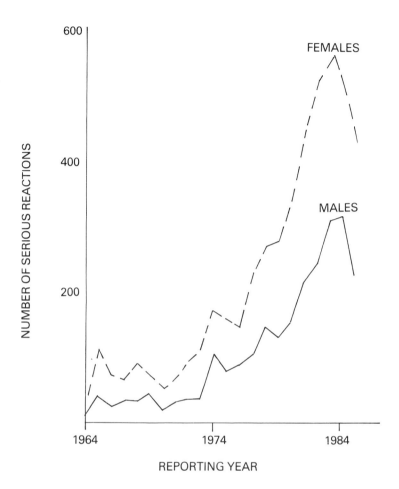

Figure 9 Serious adverse reactions associated with NSAIDs in the years 1964–1985. Males: solid line; females: dotted line

number of these reports received in the last decade can be seen in the figure, which is derived from data previously published[38].

A number of NSAIDs have been withdrawn from clinical use for reasons which have included their unacceptable adverse reactions experience. Nine of these withdrawn drugs are shown in Table 4, which presents a classification of this group of drugs by chemical type. It is perhaps disturbing that the withdrawn drugs are members of the

Table 4   Non–steroidal anti-inflammatory drugs

1. **Salicylates**
   Aspirin
   Benorylate
   Diflunisal
   Aloxiprin
   Salsalate
   Trilisate

2. **Arylalkanoic acids**
   Phenylpropionic acid derivates
   Benoxaprofen★
   Ibuprofen
   Indoprofen★
   Ketoprofen
   Flurbiprofen
   Fenoprofen
   Fenbufen
   Suprofen★

   Naphthylpropionic acid derivatives
   Naproxen

   Phenylacetic acid derivatives
   Fenclofenac★
   Diclofenac
   Alclofenac★
   Ibufenac

3. **Anthranilic acids**
   Mefenamic acid
   Flufenamic acid★

4. **Pyrazolones**
   Phenylbutazone†
   Oxyphenbutazone★
   Azapropazone
   Feprazone★

5. **Cyclic acetic acids**
   Indomethacin
   (Osmosin brand of indomethacin★)
   Sulindac
   Tolmetin
   Zomepirac★

6. **Oxicams**
   Piroxicam

★Withdrawn from use; †restricted in use

arylalkanoic acids, the anthranilic acids, the pyrazolones and the cyclic acetic acids — in other words, from a wide range of chemical types of NSAIDs. This must suggest that the underlying pharmacological mode of action of this class of drug is associated with clinical toxicity. In addition to the withdrawn drugs shown in Table 4, phenylbutazone has been restricted in use to the management of ankylosing spondylitis treated in hospitals.

A certain amount of information[40] has become available regarding some of these withdrawn NSAIDs. Table 5 relates prescription volume to marketing period and the number of yellow card reports in respect of benoxaprofen, zomepirac, Osmosin (the special slow-release form of indomethacin), and indoprofen. The data in Table 5 do not reflect all the issues taken into account at the time when these drugs were withdrawn. They do, however, suggest that the marketing life of drugs of this type which are withdrawn is quite short — less than two years. Additionally, the number of prescriptions is fairly limited — less than 1.5 million. It may be that these two factors vaguely define the range which must be covered by postmarketing surveillance studies designed to cover the difficult safety evaluation period which follows the Product Licence stage (based, usually, on data from about 3000 or so patients) and precedes the time when experience is so extensive that, about three or five years after marketing, the drug loses its "black triangle" in the British National Formulary.

Despite these drug withdrawals, seven of the ten drugs most frequently reported as the suspected cause of serious adverse reactions

Table 5   Marketing period and prescription volume with four withdrawn NSAIDs

Drug	Marketing period (months)*	Reports †	Deaths †	Prescriptions *	Prescriptions for one report	Prescriptions for one death
Benoxaprofen	22	4 086	89	1 500 000	367	16 854
Zomepirac	23	602	8	900 000	1 495	112 500
Osmosin‡	10	717	36	400 000	558	11 111
Indoprofen	12	269	10	120 000	446	12 000

*From Mann[40]
†From CSM FO6S print-out run on 3rd July 1986
‡Brand of indomethacin

are NSAIDs. The ten drugs and the number of serious adverse reaction reports for the period January to June 1986 are shown in Table 6. It must be appreciated that many of the drugs shown in this table are massively prescribed and the number of reports, even of serious suspected reactions, must reflect, amongst other factors, the degree of use of a drug as well as its apparent clinical toxicity.

Profiles of the NSAIDs

It will be remembered that the Committee on Safety of Medicines[39] concluded that the adverse reaction profile of the individual NSAIDs varies. This observation is of special interest for it is possible that the adverse reaction profile might reflect the chemical structure or pharmacological properties of the individual drug. This might be the darker side of a mirror in which the brighter possibilities of structure activity relationships have been observed for some time.

To consider this possibility the FO6S computer summaries of the Committee on Safety of Medicines have been examined. These each relate to one drug only and summarise the reactions reported in which the designated drug is the suspect cause. The reports list only the most important adverse reaction in the individual patient (MIREA). Thus the total number of reports listed in the FO6S for a drug equals the

Table 6   The ten drugs most frequently reported as the suspected cause of serious adverse reactions

Number of serious adverse reaction reports	Suspected drug, January–June 1986
100	Piroxicam
80	Fenbufen
78	Enalapril maleate
77	Naproxen
59	Diclofenac sodium
52	Indomethacin
44	Co-trimoxazole
41	Ibuprofen
41	Ketoprofen
39	Captopril
611	

total number of yellow cards received in respect of that drug, even though some patients may have suffered more than one adverse reaction. The summaries are subject to the minor inexactitudes of data collected over long periods of time and individual reports seldom establish causality, especially when concomitant medication has been given in the individual patient.

Certain types of adverse reactions dominate the clinical picture in respect of the NSAIDs and special attention has been paid to reactions which, for one or other of the individual NSAIDs, account for 5% or more of the total reports noted on the FO6S. These types of reactions comprise nail disorder, photosensitivity, rash, urticaria, headache, gastrointestinal intolerance, gastrointestinal haemorrhage, gastro-intestinal perforation, hepatitis (including major abnormalities of hepatic function) and jaundice, aplastic anaemia (including marrow aplasia and depression and pancytopenia), agranulocytosis (including granulocytopenia and leucopenia), thrombocytopenia, nephritis (including major degrees of renal function abnormality, nephropathy and renal papillary necrosis) and anaphylaxis (including major allergic reactions and anaphylactoid reactions). Other individual reactions, for the different drugs, account for less than 5% of the total noted on the FO6S. Thus, in many instances, they reflect small numbers of reports in which the causal relationship to the drug is exceptionally difficult to evaluate. In this analysis, the term "gastrointestinal intoler-ance" represents the sum of the reports for abdominal pain, diarrhoea, dyspepsia, nausea and vomiting.

Examining the drugs in this way has the advantage that one is concerned only with the percentage of reports (or fatal reports) due to different types of reactions. It is informative, provided the number of reports is large enough to make consideration of percentage values acceptable and provided it is kept in mind that percentage values for common effects with a drug may dwarf the impression given of an uncommon effect even when that effect is, though relatively infrequent, of great clinical importance. The major bias would appear to be differential reporting of one type of reaction, so distorting the picture. Piroxicam, for instance, has been so widely spoken of as a drug which may cause gastrointestinal bleeds that such bleeds in patients receiving piroxicam might be reported when they would remain unreported with other drugs. Another bias may arise from gross under-reporting; this might make the ratio of reports due to the different types of adverse effect almost arbitrary as a small-number phenomenon.

Such biases would seem most likely to distort the profile of aspirin, as this drug was introduced into clinical practice in 1899. In fact, as is evident from Table 7 and Figure 10, the FO6S for acetylsalicylic acid shows a very characteristic NSAID profile. 192 (47.5%) of the total of 404 reports and 67 (74.5%) of the 90 fatal reports included within the total were due to gastrointestinal haemorrhage. Twenty (5.0%) of the reports were due to urticaria (and this was the only non-gastrointestinal type of reaction causing 5% or more of the reports); however,

Table 7   Adverse reactions profile for acetylsalicylic acid

	Reports		Deaths	
	Number	*%*	*Number*	*%*
Nail disorder	0	0	0	0
Photosensitivity	0	0	0	0
Rash	16	4.0	0	0
Urticaria	20	5.0	0	0
Headache	4	1.0	0	0
Gastrointestinal intolerance	8	2.0	0	0
Gastrointestinal haemorrhage	192	47.5	67	74.5
Gastrointestinal perforation	6	1.5	4	4.4
Hepatitis, disordered hepatic function, jaundice, etc.	5	1.2	1	1.1
Aplastic anaemia, marrow aplasia and depression, pancytopenia, etc.	1	0.2	0	0
Agranulocytosis, granulocytopenia, leucopenia, etc.	1	0.2	1	1.1
Thrombocytopenia	6	1.5	0	0
Nephritis, disordered renal function, nephropathy, renal papillary necrosis, etc.	12	3.0	7	7.8
Anaphylaxis, allergic and anaphylactoid reactions	10	2.5	1	1.1
Others	123	30.4	9	10.0
Total	404	100.0	90	100.0

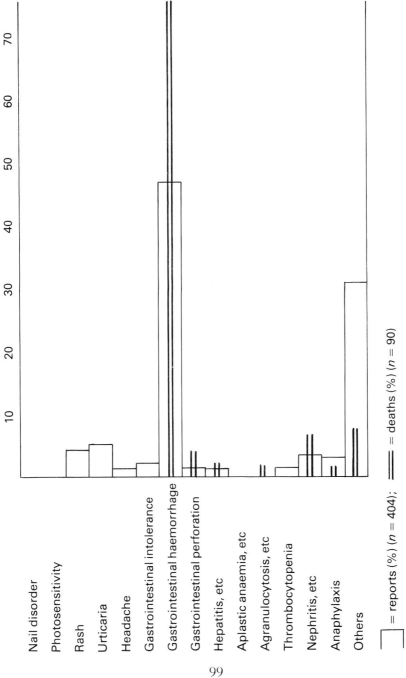

Nail disorder

Photosensitivity

Rash

Urticaria

Headache

Gastrointestinal intolerance

Gastrointestinal haemorrhage

Gastrointestinal perforation

Hepatitis, etc

Aplastic anaemia, etc

Agranulocytosis, etc

Thrombocytopenia

Nephritis, etc

Anaphylaxis

Others

☐ = reports (%) (*n* = 404);   ▦ = deaths (%) (*n* = 90)

Figure 10   Adverse reactions — acetylsalicylic acid

a notable 12 (3.0%) of the reports were due to angioedema, and 11 (2.7%) were due to asthma. Seven (7.8%) of the 90 deaths were due to thrombocytopenia. Thus, despite presumed gross under-reporting, doctors sometimes report troublesome adverse effects which seem related to the use of acetylsalicylic acid. The extreme rarity of these effects, apart perhaps from gastrointestinal haemorrhage, must serve as a reminder that no active drug is totally devoid of unwanted effects.

Ibuprofen, previously noted as one of the possibly safer NSAIDs at the doses used in the past, also has a typical NSAID profile in that most of the deaths in which it has been the suspect drug have been due to gastrointestinal haemorrhage. The data are summarised in Table 8 and illustrated in Figure 11. Compared with other drugs in the series

Table 8   Adverse reactions profile for ibuprofen

	Reports		Deaths	
	Number	*%*	*Number*	*%*
Nail disorder	7	0.4	0	0
Photosensitivity	17	1.0	0	0
Rash	167	9.9	0	0
Urticaria	58	3.5	0	0
Headache	18	1.0	0	0
Gastrointestinal intolerance	110	6.6	0	0
Gastrointestinal haemorrhage	216	12.9	22	41.5
Gastrointestinal perforation	27	1.6	9	17.0
Hepatitis, disordered hepatic function, jaundice, etc.	29	1.7	1	1.9
Aplastic anaemia, marrow aplasia and depression, pancytopenia, etc.	25	1.5	12	22.6
Agranulocytosis, granulocytopenia, leucopenia, etc.	28	1.7	1	1.9
Thrombocytopenia	58	3.5	2	3.8
Nephritis, disordered renal function, nephropathy, renal papillary necrosis, etc.	14	0.8	0	0
Anaphylaxis, allergic and anaphylactoid reactions	17	1.0	0	0
Others	888	52.9	6	11.3
Total	1679	100.0	53	100.0

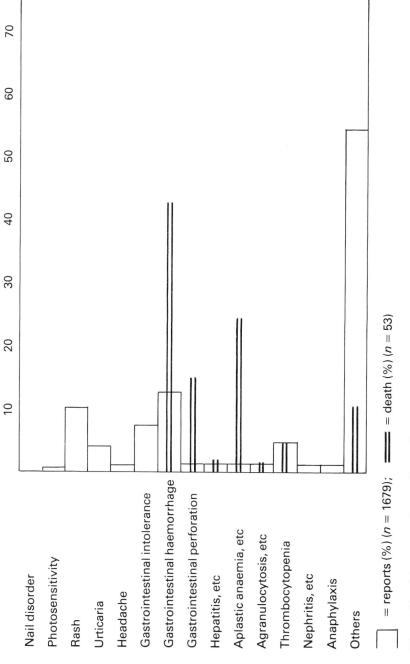

Figure 11 Adverse reactions — ibuprofen

☐ = reports (%) (*n* = 1679);   ▦ = death (%) (*n* = 53)

the profile is mild and 888 (52.9%) of the 1679 reports arise from reactions other than those characteristic of the NSAIDs. The deaths, despite the enormous use of the drug, amount to only 53: 22 (41.5%) of these were due to gastrointestinal bleeds, 9 (17.0%) were due to gut perforation, and 12 (22.6%) resulted from aplastic anaemia. Amongst the reports, 78 (4.6%) were due to angioedema and 64 (3.8%) to asthma.

Naproxen (Table 9 and Figure 12) and indomethacin, even when including Osmosin, (Table 10 and Figure 13) have somewhat similar profiles, though the proportions of gastrointestinal haemorrhages are a little larger than with ibuprofen. There have been 1926 reports, including 94 fatal reports, with naproxen and no less than 3135, including 274 fatal reports, with indomethacin. Both drugs, like

Table 9 Adverse reactions profile for naproxen

	Reports		Deaths	
	Number	*%*	*Number*	*%*
Nail disorder	5	0.3	0	0
Photosensitivity	41	2.1	0	0
Rash	175	9.1	0	0
Urticaria	71	3.7	0	0
Headache	21	1.1	0	0
Gastrointestinal intolerance	154	8.0	0	0
Gastrointestinal haemorrhage	388	20.1	47	50.0
Gastrointestinal perforation	41	2.1	13	13.8
Hepatitis, disordered hepatic function, jaundice, etc.	28	1.6	1	1.1
Aplastic anaemia, marrow aplasia and depression, pancytopenia, etc.	22	1.1	13	13.8
Agranulocytosis, granulocytopenia, leucopenia, etc.	31	1.6	2	2.1
Thrombocytopenia	35	1.8	3	3.2
Nephritis, disordered renal function, nephropathy, renal papillary necrosis, etc.	17	0.9	3	3.2
Anaphylaxis, allergic and anaphylactoid reactions	22	1.1	0	0
Others	875	45.4	12	12.8
Total	1926	100.0	94	100.0

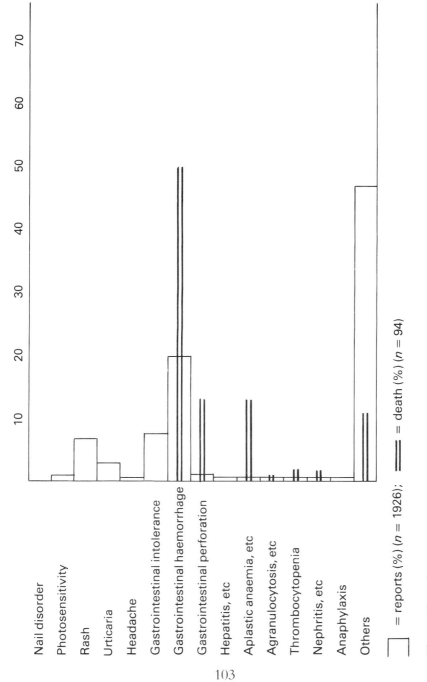

□ = reports (%) (*n* = 1926);   ▥ = death (%) (*n* = 94)

Figure 12   Adverse reactions — naproxen

ibuprofen, are associated with reports of angioedema and asthma: 77 (4.0%) of the naproxen reports show angioedema as the most important reaction, whilst 46 (2.4%) relate to asthma. Angioedema produced 28 (0.9%) of the reports with indomethacin and asthma was the most important reaction in 30 (1.0%) of the reports with this drug. Indomethacin is known to produce headache and 259 (8.3%) of the reports with this drug were due to this cause.

The Committee on Safety of Medicines[41] noted that Osmosin was associated with a high rate of reporting and with reports of intestinal perforation distal to the duodenum — an unusual site for damage associated with a non-steroidal anti-inflammatory agent.

Some of the NSAIDs have an adverse reactions profile which is rather obviously different from the typical pattern. Fenbufen and

Table 10   Adverse reactions profile for indomethacin

	Reports		Deaths	
	Number	%	Number	%
Nail disorder	6	0.2	0	0
Photosensitivity	16	0.5	0	0
Rash	91	2.9	0	0
Urticaria	41	1.3	0	0
Headache	259	8.3	0	0
Gastrointestinal intolerance	340	10.8	1	0.4
Gastrointestinal haemorrhage	480	15.3	126	46.0
Gastrointestinal perforation	183	5.8	60	21.9
Hepatitis, disordered hepatic function, jaundice, etc.	56	1.8	11	4.0
Aplastic anaemia, marrow aplasia and depression, pancytopenia, etc.	50	1.6	22	8.0
Agranulocytosis, granulocytopenia, leucopenia, etc.	33	1.1	8	2.9
Thrombocytopenia	61	2.0	4	1.5
Nephritis, disordered renal function, nephropathy, renal papillary necrosis, etc.	23	0.7	3	1.1
Anaphylaxis, allergic and anaphylactoid reactions	7	0.2	0	0
Others	1489	47.5	39	14.2
Total	3135	100.0	274	100.0

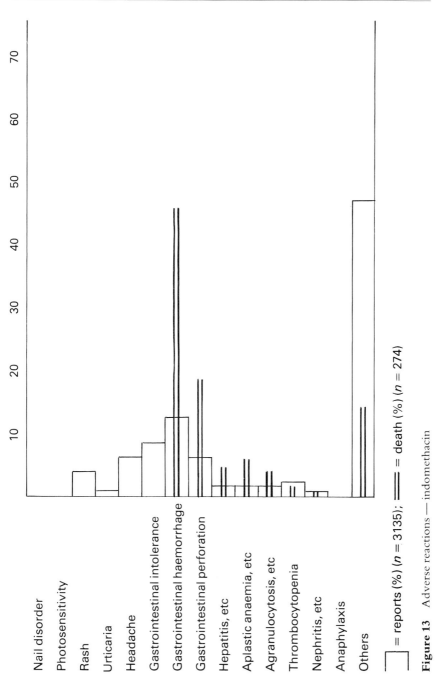

Figure 13   Adverse reactions — indomethacin

☐ = reports (%) (n = 3135);   ▦ = death (%) (n = 274)

benoxaprofen, for example, are associated with a disproportionately large number of reports of skin reactions; phenylbutazone and oxyphenbutazone cause, or certainly appear to cause, a large number of blood dyscrasias, and piroxicam has a profile which is so dominated by gastrointestinal haemorrhage as to be remarkable.

The information on fenbufen is summarised in Table 11 and Figure 14. Of the 4495 reports which have been received, no less than 2747 (61.1%) are concerned with rashes and another 457 (10.2%) with urticaria. These cutaneous responses are not always mild or moderate in severity and there have been 130 (2.3%) reports of erythema multiforme and 52 (1.6%) reports of purpura or purpuric rashes. Yet only 17 of these 4495 reports have been concerned with fatalities.

The situation was very different with benoxaprofen (Table 12 and

Table 11   Adverse reactions profile for fenbufen

	Reports		Deaths	
	Number	%	Number	%
Nail disorder	4	0.1	0	0
Photosensitivity	53	1.2	0	0
Rash	2747	61.1	0	0
Urticaria	457	10.2	0	0
Headache	36	0.8	0	0
Gastrointestinal intolerance	262	5.8	0	0
Gastrointestinal haemorrhage	89	2.0	2	11.8
Gastrointestinal perforation	4	0.1	2	11.8
Hepatitis, disordered hepatic function, jaundice, etc.	23	0.5	0	0
Aplastic anaemia, marrow aplasia and depression, pancytopenia, etc.	13	0.3	4	23.5
Agranulocytosis, granulocytopenia, leucopenia, etc.	12	0.3	1	5.9
Thrombocytopenia	11	0.2	0	0
Nephritis, disordered renal function, nephropathy, renal papillary necrosis, etc.	10	0.2	2	11.8
Anaphylaxis, allergic and anaphylactoid reactions	26	0.6	0	0
Others	748	16.6	6	35.2
Total	4495	100.0	17	100.0

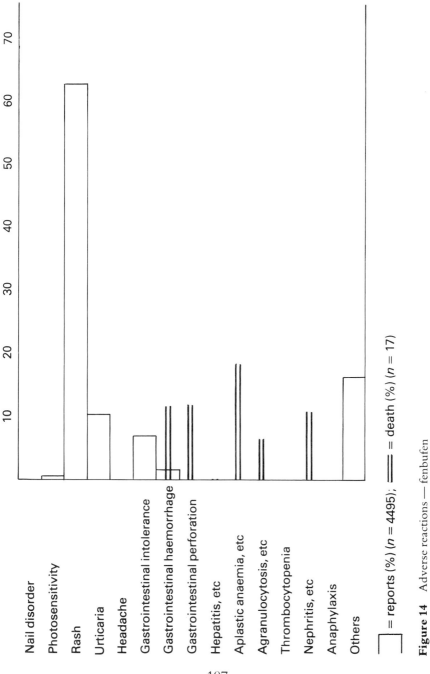

Nail disorder
Photosensitivity
Rash
Urticaria
Headache
Gastrointestinal intolerance
Gastrointestinal haemorrhage
Gastrointestinal perforation
Hepatitis, etc
Aplastic anaemia, etc
Agranulocytosis, etc
Thrombocytopenia
Nephritis, etc
Anaphylaxis
Others

□ = reports (%) (*n* = 4495);   ▤ = death (%) (*n* = 17)

Figure 14   Adverse reactions — fenbufen

Figure 15). There were 4086 reports and 89 of these were concerned with fatalities. The pattern of the reports was quite different from the deaths, and this is itself unusual. The reports were dominated by skin reactions: 364 (8.9%) related to nail disorders, no less than 1545 (37.8%) related to photosensitivity, 677 (16.6%) related to rash, and in 127 (3.1%) urticaria was thought to be the most important reaction. None of the fatalities arose from these cutaneous reactions. From that point of view, benoxaprofen might have looked like fenbufen: a drug associated with a great number of reports but most of these skin reactions, none of which were lethal. The pattern of the 89 deaths as shown on the computer record is different: gastrointestinal bleeds and perforations yielded only 19 reports in which the outcome was death.

Table 12   Adverse reactions profile for benoxaprofen

	Reports		Deaths	
	Number	%	Number	%
Nail disorder	364	8.9	0	0
Photosensitivity	1545	37.8	0	0
Rash	677	16.6	0	0
Urticaria	127	3.1	0	0
Headache	27	0.7	0	0
Gastrointestinal intolerance	173	4.2	0	0
Gastrointestinal haemorrhage	98	2.4	7	7.9
Gastrointestinal perforation	15	0.4	12	13.5
Hepatitis, disordered hepatic function, jaundice, etc.	105	2.6	33	37.1
Aplastic anaemia, marrow aplasia and depression, pancytopenia, etc.	18	0.4	7	7.9
Agranulocytosis, granulocytopenia, leucopenia, etc.	16	0.4	4	4.5
Thrombocytopenia	37	0.9	2	2.2
Nephritis, disordered renal function, nephropathy, renal papillary necrosis, etc.	25	0.6	10	11.2
Anaphylaxis, allergic and anaphylactoid reactions	10	0.2	0	0
Others	849	20.8	14	15.7
Total	4086	100.0	89	100.0

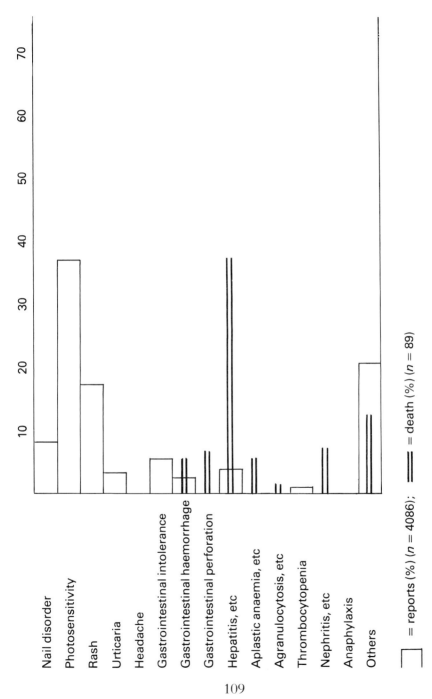

Figure 15 Adverse reactions — benoxaprofen

□ = reports (%) (*n* = 4086);   ▐▐ = death (%) (*n* = 89)

However, 33 (37.1%) of the 89 fatal reports were concerned with hepatic lesions as the most important reaction in the individual subject. Ten (11.2%) of the fatal reactions concerned renal disorders and 7 (7.9%) of the 89 fatalities occurred in patients with aplastic anaemia or loosely related conditions. Benoxaprofen, then, came to be recognised as a drug with a malign profile and the fatal reports included a hepato-renal syndrome and a number of blood dyscrasias. That there were remarkably few cases of major gastrointestinal disorders with this drug did not save it from withdrawal due to its adverse reactions profile.

The outline of the profile of phenylbutazone is given in Table 13 and Figure 16. There were relatively few reports for skin reactions with this drug but there were some gastrointestinal bleeds: these accounted

Table 13   Adverse reactions profile for phenylbutazone

	Reports		Deaths	
	Number	%	Number	%
Nail disorder	1	0.1	0	0
Photosensitivity	4	0.2	0	0
Rash	154	9.0	0	0
Urticaria	33	1.9	0	0
Headache	8	0.5	0	0
Gastrointestinal intolerance	29	1.7	0	0
Gastrointestinal haemorrhage	206	12.0	63	14.0
Gastrointestinal perforation	29	1.7	9	2.0
Hepatitis, disordered hepatic function, jaundice, etc.	67	3.9	7	1.6
Aplastic anaemia, marrow aplasia and depression, pancytopenia, etc.	370	21.5	245	54.6
Agranulocytosis, granulocytopenia, leucopenia, etc.	107	6.2	43	9.6
Thrombocytopenia	73	4.2	19	4.2
Nephritis, disordered renal function, nephropathy, renal papillary necrosis, etc.	18	1.0	3	0.6
Anaphylaxis, allergic and anaphylactoid reactions	1	0.1	0	0
Others	619	36.0	60	13.4
Total	1719	100.0	449	100.0

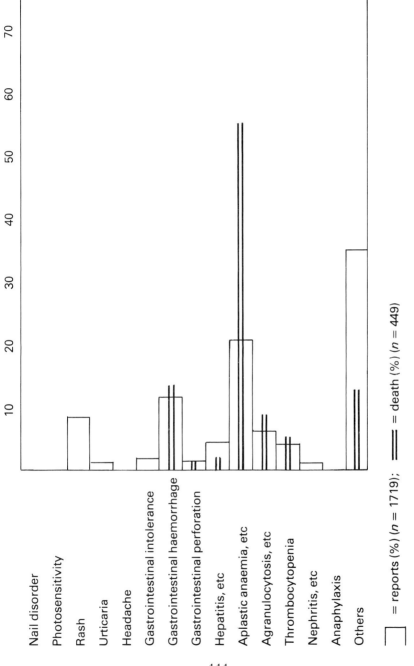

Figure 16 Adverse reactions — phenylbutazone

☐ = reports (%) (*n* = 1719); ▮▮ = death (%) (*n* = 449)

for 206 (12.0%) of the total of 1719 reports and for 63 (14.0%) of the 449 deaths. However, the profile, both in terms of total reports and those reports within the total which were concerned with fatalities, was dominated by blood dyscrasias. 370 (21.5%) of the reports and 245 (54.6%) of the deaths arose from aplastic anaemia or conditions of that type. That this slowly mounting total of fatal reports was tolerated for so long indicates the vast use and usefulness of this drug, which is now much restricted in use. Oxyphenbutazone, which produced a comparable adverse reactions picture, has now been totally withdrawn from use.

Piroxicam (Table 14 and Figure 17) again has a rather unique adverse reactions profile, which is of special interest as the drug is the first of its chemical type to enter widespread clinical use. There have been a

Table 14   Adverse reactions profile for piroxicam

	Reports		Deaths	
	Number	%	Number	%
Nail disorder	23	0.8	0	0
Photosensitivity	95	3.5	0	0
Rash	299	11.0	0	0
Urticaria	72	2.6	0	0
Headache	29	1.1	0	0
Gastrointestinal intolerance	217	8.0	0	0
Gastrointestinal haemorrhage	612	22.5	58	59.2
Gastrointestinal perforation	124	4.6	19	19.4
Hepatitis, disordered hepatic function, jaundice, etc.	36	1.3	3	3.1
Aplastic anaemia, marrow aplasia and depression, pancytopenia, etc.	12	0.4	6	6.1
Agranulocytosis, granulocytopenia, leucopenia, etc.	8	0.7	1	1.0
Thrombocytopenia	33	1.2	0	0
Nephritis, disordered renal function, nephropathy, renal papillary necrosis, etc.	16	0.6	0	0
Anaphylaxis, allergic and anaphylactoid reactions	10	0.4	0	0
Others	1121	41.3	11	11.2
Total	2717	100.0	98	100.0

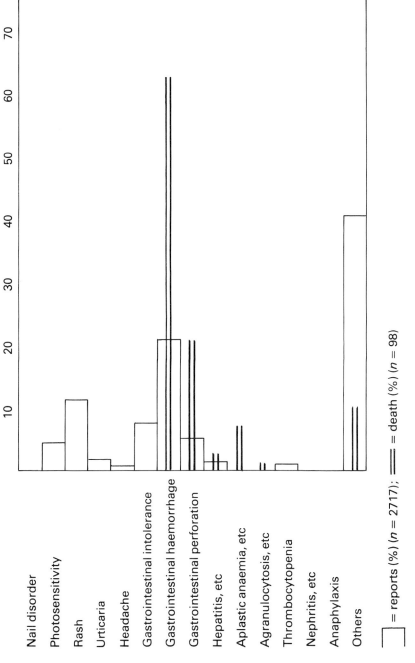

Nail disorder

Photosensitivity

Rash

Urticaria

Headache

Gastrointestinal intolerance

Gastrointestinal haemorrhage

Gastrointestinal perforation

Hepatitis, etc

Aplastic anaemia, etc

Agranulocytosis, etc

Thrombocytopenia

Nephritis, etc

Anaphylaxis

Others

☐ = reports (%) (*n* = 2717); ▥ = death (%) (*n* = 98)

Figure 17 Adverse reactions — piroxicam

relatively limited number of reports of skin reactions but a considerable proportion of reports of gastrointestinal difficulties: 612 (22.5%) of the 2717 reports and a notable 58 (59.2%) of the 98 fatal reports have been due to gastrointestinal haemorrhage. An additional 124 (4.6%) of the reports and 19 (19.4%) of the deaths have been due to gastrointestinal perforation. Another, even though minor, feature of the drug is that 118 (4.3%) of the reports have been due to oedema and 27 (1.0%) have concerned cardiac failure.

Conclusion

The yellow card system serves principally as an alerting mechanism and the data so far available clearly indicate that the non-steroidal anti-inflammatory drugs are, as a group, an important cause of serious adverse reactions. This impression has been confirmed by clinical studies such as those of Walt and colleagues (1986)[42] and Armstrong and Blower (1987)[43]. It has received important confirmation from the case-control study of Somerville, Faulkner and Langman (1986)[44]. Nevertheless, the literature remains conflicting and, in the absence of a number of case-control studies of adequate size, action in the public interest has had to be taken by either the regulatory bodies or the companies concerned in respect of the drugs which appeared to offer markedly greater risks for the degree of benefit conferred. It seems clear that a number of special types of study, including a number of large case-control studies, are essential if the NSAIDs now remaining on the market are to be ranked to secure the most favourable benefit to risk ratio. Such studies are also needed in order to determine whether these drugs are appropriate in relatively trivial indications for use, whether the currently used doses are optimal, and whether there are vulnerable age- or sex-related groups in whom these drugs should be contra-indicated except in the presence of disease which is non-responsive to other remedies and of such severity that fairly sizeable risks are considered acceptable. The need for these studies defines our current research objectives, which are:

(1) To determine whether one of the drugs still on the market is less safe than the others.

(2) To determine whether the use of the NSAIDs should be restricted to serious disease.
(3) To secure use of the lowest effective dose.
(4) To lessen or exclude use in any specially vulnerable groups of patients.

In the light of the valuable comments of Lord Justice Lawton[45], studies of the type envisaged are probably essential before valid informed consent can be obtained for the use of prescription-only NSAIDs in patients with the less serious or trivial degrees of disease.

These general conclusions do, of course, exclude certain specific issues which relate to one drug only of the NSAID series. An example of such an issue is the relationship of Reye's syndrome to the use of aspirin[46,47] in children. The present concern is with the use of NSAIDs in the treatment of pain and painful conditions.

Typically the NSAIDs are associated with a large number of reports of skin, gastrointestinal, and haematological adverse reactions (suggesting that they challenge the organ systems in which the body cells replicate most frequently); they also produce comparatively large numbers of reports of hepatic and renal adverse reactions (suggesting that they adversely affect the organs of metabolic activity and excretion). Whilst there is this characteristic pattern of adverse reactions to the NSAIDs — and it is an unhappy picture — it is evident that the profile of some of these drugs varies markedly from that typical of the drug class. The tendency for the pyrazolones to cause blood dyscrasias of a number of types seems well marked — azapropazone, apart from haemolytic anaemia and related changes, may be something of an exception. Fenbufen and benoxaprofen typify those NSAIDs which are associated with a large proportion of reports of skin reactions; both are phenylpropionic acid derivatives — but others of this chemical group show this characteristic to a less marked extent. In view of the profile of piroxicam and the number of reports of serious gastrointestinal reactions associated with this drug, additions to the range of oxicams will need to be watched very carefully upon introduction into clinical use.

Because the profile of these drugs does vary it may be possible to produce NSAIDs synthesised so as to avoid molecular features or pharmacological attributes which seem to be associated with particular unwanted adverse effects. The attempts to define such relationships between chemical, pharmacological or pharmacokinetic features and clinical toxicity represent a further research objective and such studies are in progress.

References

1. Mann, R. D. (1984). *Modern Drug Use, an Enquiry on Historical Principles*, pp 268–70. Lancaster and Boston: MTP Press
2. Markham, C. R. (1874). *A Memoir of the Lady Ana de Osorio, Countess of Chinchon and Vice-Queen of Peru (AD 1629–39) with a Plea for the Correct Spelling of the Chinchona Genus.* London: Trübner
3. Runge, F. F. (1834). Ueber einige Produkte der Steinkohlen-destillation. *Ann. Phys. Chem. (Lpz.)* (Poggendorff's Annal), **31**, 65–78, 513–24; **32**, 308–33
4. Lemaire, F. J. (1860). Du Coaltar Saponiné, Désinfectant Énergique, Arrétant les Fermentations. Paris: Germer Baillière
5. Lister, J., 1st Baron Lister (1867). On a new method of treating compound fracture, abscess, etc., with observations on the conditions of suppuration. *Lancet*, **1**, 326–9, 357–9, 387–9, 507–9; **2**, 95–6
6. Lister, J., 1st Baron Lister (1867). On the antiseptic principle in the practice of surgery. *Lancet*, **2**, 353–6, 668–9
7. Knorr, L. (1884). Üeber die Constitution der Chinizin-derivate. *Chem. Berl.*, **17**, 2032–49
8. Filehne, W. (1884). Ueber das Antipyrin, ein neues Antipyreticum. *Zeit. klin. Med.*, **7**, 641–2
9. Filehne, W. (1896). Ueber das Pyramidon, ein Antipyrinderivat. *Berl. klin. Wschr.*, **33**, 1061–3
10. Rechenberg, von H. K. (ed.) (1962). *Butazolidin (Phenylbutazone).* London: Arnold
11. Martindale, W. (1977). In Wade, A. and Reynolds, J. E. F. (eds) *The Extra Pharmacopoeia, Incorporating Squire's Companion*, 27th edn, p. 187. London: The Pharmaceutical Press
12. Martindale, W. (1977). In Wade, A. and Reynolds, J. E. F. (eds)

The Extra Pharmacopoeia, Incorporating Squire's Companion, 27th edn, p. 208. London: The Pharmaceutical Press

13. Leviticus 23:40. *The Bible* (Authorised Version)

14. British Pharmaceutical Codex (1934). *The British Pharmaceutical Codex 1934, an Imperial Dispensatory for the Use of Medical Practitioners and Pharmacists*, pp 918–19. London: The Pharmaceutical Press

15. Leake, C. D. (1975). *An Historical Account of Pharmacology to the Twentieth Century*, p. 160. Springfield, Illinois: Charles C. Thomas

16. Stone, Rev. E. (1763). An account of the success of the bark of the willow in the cure of agues. *Philosophical Transactions, Giving Some Account of the Present Undertakings, Studies, and Labours, of the Ingenious, in Many Considerable Parts of the World*, **53**, 195–200

17. James, S. (1792). *Observations on the Bark of a Particular Species of Willow, Showing its Superiority to the Peruvian and its Singular Efficacy in the Cure of Agues, etc.* London: Johnson

18. White, W. (1798). *Observations and Experiments on the Broad-Leaved Willow Bark, Illustrated with Cases.* Bath: Hazard

19. Wilkinson, G. (1803). *Experiments and Observations on the Cortex Salicis Latifoliae or Broad-Leaved Willow Bark.* Newcastle-upon-Tyne: Walker

20. British Pharmaceutical Codex (1934). *The British Pharmaceutical Codex 1934, an Imperial Dispensatory for the Use of Medical Practitioners and Pharmacists*, pp 917–18. London: The Pharmaceutical Press

21. Leroux, H. (1830). *J. Chim. Méd.*, **6**, 340–2

22. Piria, R. (1839). Recherches sur la Salicine et les produits qui en dérivent. *C. R. Acad. Sci. (Paris)*, **8**, 479–85

23. Gerland, H. (1852). New formation of salicylic acid. *J. Chem. Soc.*, **5**, 133–8

24. Buss, C. E. (1875). Ueber die Anwendung der Salicylsäure als Antipyreticum. *Dtsch. Arch. klin. Med.*, **15**, 457–501

25. Maclagan, T. (1876). The treatment of acute rheumatism by salicin. *Lancet*, **1**, 342–3

26. Maclagan, T. (1876). The treatment of rheumatism by salicin and salicylic acid. *Br. Med. J.*, **1**, 627

27. Stricker, S. (1876). Ueber die Resultate der Behandlung der Poly-arthritis rheumatica mit Salicylsäure. *Berl. klin. Wschr.*, **13**, 99–103

28. Gerhardt, C. F. (1853). Untersuchungen über die wasserfreien organischen Säuren. *Leibig's Ann.*, **87**, 149–79

29. Dreser, H. (1899). Pharmakologisches über Aspirin (Acetylsali-cylsäure). *Pflüg. Arch. ges. Physiol.*, **76**, 306–18

30. Sneader, W. (1985). *Drug Discovery: The Evolution of Modern Medicines*, p. 82. Chichester, New York, Brisbane, Toronto and Singapore: John Wiley and Sons

31. Witthauer, K. (1899). Aspirin, ein neues Salicylpreparat. *Die Heilkunde*, **3**, 396

32. Winder, C. V., Wax, J., Scotti, L., Scherrer, R. A., Jones, E. M. and Short, F. W. (1962). Anti-inflammatory, antipyretic and antinociceptive properties of N-(2,3-xylyl) anthranilic acid (mefenamic acid). *J. Pharm. Exp. Ther.*, **138**, 405–13

33. Shen, T. Y., Windholz, T. B., Rosegay, A., Witzel, B. E., Wilson, A. N., Willett, J. D., Holtz, W. J., Ellis, R. L., Matzuk, A. R., Lucas, S., Stammer, C. H., Holly, F. W., Sarett, L. H., Risley, E. A., Nuss, G. W. and Winter, C. A. (1963). Non-steroid anti-inflammatory agents. *J. Am. Chem. Soc.*, **85**, 488–9

34. Nicholson, J. S. (1982). Ibuprofen. In Bindra, J. S. and Lednicer, D. (eds) *Chronicles of Drug Discovery*, Vol. 1, pp 149–72. Chiches-ter: John Wiley

35. Wiseman, E. H. and Lombardino, J. G. (1982). Piroxicam. In Bindra, J. S. and Lednicer, D. (eds) *Chronicles of Drug Discovery*, pp 173–200. Chichester: John Wiley

36. Rodnan, G. P. and Benedek, T. G. (1970). The early history of antirheumatic drugs. *Arthritis and Rheumatism*, **13**, 145–65

37. Rainsford, K. D. (ed.) (1985). *Anti-inflammatory and Anti-rheumatic Drugs* (3 vols). Boca Raton, Florida: CRC Press

38. Mann, R. D. (1987). The yellow card data: the nature and scale of the adverse drug reactions problem. In Mann, R. D. (ed.) *Adverse Drug Reactions, the Scale and Nature of the Problem and the Way Forward*, pp 5–66. Carnforth and New Jersey: Parthenon Publishing

39. Committee on Safety of Medicines (1986). CSM update: Non-steroidal anti-inflammatory drugs and serious gastrointestinal

adverse reactions – 2. *Brit. Med. J.*, **292**, 1190–1

40. Mann, R. D. (1984). *Modern Drug Use, an Enquiry on Historical Principles*, pp 709–12. Lancaster and Boston: MTP Press

41. Committee on Safety of Medicines (1983). *Current Problems*, No. 11, August 1983. London: H.M.S.O.

42. Walt, R., Logan, R., Katschinski, B., Ashley, J. and Langman, M. (1986). Rising frequency of ulcer perforation in elderly people in the United Kingdom. *Lancet*, **1**, 489–92

43. Armstrong, C. P. and Blower, A. L. (1987). Non-steroidal anti-inflammatory drugs and life threatening complications of peptic ulceration. *Gut*, **28**, 527–32

44. Somerville, K., Faulkner, G. and Langman, M. (1986). Non-steroidal anti-inflammatory drugs and bleeding peptic ulcer. *Lancet*, **1**, 462–4

45. Lawton, The Right Hon. Lord Justice (1983). Legal aspects of iatrogenic disorders: discussion paper. *J. Roy. Soc. Med.*, **76**, 289–91

46. Committee on Safety of Medicines (1986). CSM update: Reye's Syndrome and aspirin. *Br. Med. J.*, **292**, 1590

47. Mann, R. D. (1986). Reye's Syndrome and aspirin. *J. Roy. Coll. Gen. Pract.*, **36**, 418–21

Editor's note

The figures for fenbufen in Table 2 (page 90) were revised (Cohen, P. and Mann, R. D. (1986), *Br. Med. J.*, **293**, 51) to give prescriptions (million) of 1.97; total serious reactions per million prescriptions 55.3 (3.6), serious gastrointestinal reactions per million prescriptions 28.4 (1.5), other serious reactions per million prescriptions 26.9 (2.0).

Appendix 1

[195]

XXXII. *An Account of the Succe/s of the Bark of the Willow in the Cure of Agues. In a Letter to the Right Honourable* George *Earl of* Macclesfield, *Prefident of R. S. from the Rev. Mr.* Edmund Stone, *of* Chipping-Norton *in* Oxfordfhire.

My Lord,

Read June 2d, 1763.
A Mong the many ufeful difcoveries, which this age hath made, there are very few which, better deferve the attention of the public than what I am going to lay before your Lordfhip.

There is a bark of an Englifh tree, which I have found by experience to be a powerful aftringent, and very efficacious in curing aguifh and intermitting diforders.

About fix years ago, I accidentally tafted it, and was furprifed at its extraordinary bitternefs; which immediately raifed me a fufpicion of its having the properties of the Peruvian bark. As this tree delights in a moift or wet foil, where agues chiefly abound, the general maxim, that many natural maladies carry their cures along with them, or that their remedies lie not far from their caufes, was fo very appofite to this particular cafe, that I could not help applying it; and that this might be the intention of Providence here, I muft own had fome little weight with me.

The exceffive plenty of this bark furnifhed me, in my fpeculative difquifitions upon it, with an

D d 2   argument

[196]

argument both for and againſt theſe imaginary qualities of it ; for, on one hand, as intermittents are
very common, it was reaſonable to ſuppoſe, that what
was deſigned for their cure, ſhould be as common and
as eaſy to be procured. But then, on the other hand,
it ſeemed probable, that, if there was any conſiderable
virtue in this bark, it muſt have been diſcovered from
its plenty. My curioſity prompted me to look into
into the diſpenſatories and books of botany, and ex-
amine what they ſaid concerning it; but there it ex-
iſted only by name. I could not find, that it hath, or
ever had, any place in pharmacy, or any ſuch qualities,
as I ſuſpected aſcribed to it by the botaniſts.

However, I determined to make ſome experiments
with it; and, for this purpoſe, I gathered that ſummer
near a pound weight of it, which I dryed in a bag,
upon the outſide of a baker's oven, for more than three
months, at which time it was to be reduced to a
powder, by pounding and ſifting after the manner
that other barks are pulverized.

It was not long before I had an opportunity of
making a trial of it; but, being an entire ſtranger to its
nature, I gave it in very ſmall quantities, I think it
was about twenty grains of the powder at a doſe, and
repeated it every four hours between the fits; but with
great caution and the ſtricteſt attention to its effects :
the fits were conſiderably abated, but did not entirely
ceaſe. Not perceiving the leaſt ill conſequences, I grew
bolder with it, and in a few days encreaſed the doſe
to two ſcruples, and the ague was ſoon removed.

It was then given to ſeveral others with the ſame
ſucceſs; but I found it better anſwered the intention,
when a dram of it was taken every four hours in the
intervals of the paroxiſms.

I have

121

[197]

I have continued to ufe it as a remedy for agues and intermitting diforders for five years fucceffively and fuccefsfully. It hath been given I believe to fifty perfons, and never failed in the cure, except in a few autumual and quartan agues, with which the patients had been long and feverely afflicted; thefe it reduced in a great degree, but did not wholly take them off; the patient, at the ufual time for the return of his fit, felt fome fmattering of his diftemper, which the inceffant repetition of thefe powders could not conquer : it feemed as if their power could reach thus far and no farther, and I did fuppofe that it would not have long continued to reach fo far, and that the diftemper would have foon returned with its priftine violence; but I did not ftay to fee the iffue : I added one fifth part of the Peruvian bark to it, and with this fmall auxiliary it totally routed its adverfary. It was found neceffary likewife, in one or two obftinate cafes, at other times of the year, to mix the fame quantity of that bark with it; but thefe were cafes where the patient went abroad imprudently, and caught cold, as a poft-chaife boy did, who, being almoft recovered from an inveterate tertian ague, would follow his bufinefs, by which means he not only neglected his powders, but, meeting with bad weather, renewed his diftemper.

One fifth part was the largeft and indeed the only proportion of the quinquina made ufe of in this compofition, and this only upon extraordinary occafions : the patient was never prepared, either by vomiting, bleeding, purging, or any medicines of a fimilar intention, for the reception of this bark, but he entered upon it abruptly and immediately, and it

was

[198]

was always given in powders, with any common vehicle, as water, tea, fmall beer and fuch like. This
was done purely to afcertain its effects; and that I
might be affured the changes wrought in the patient
could not be attributed to any other thing: though,
had there been a due preparation, the moft obftinate
intermittents would probably have yielded to this bark
without any foreign affiftance: And, by all I can
judge from five years experience of it upon a number
of perfons, it appears to be a powerful abforbent,
aftringent, and febrifuge in intermitting cafes, of the
fame nature and kind with the Peruvian bark, and to
have all its properties, though perhaps not always in
in the fame degree. It feems likewife to have this additional quality, viz. to be a fafe medicine; for I never
could perceive the leaft ill effect from it, though it
had been always given without any preparation of
the patient.

The tree, from which this bark is taken, is ftiled
by Ray, in his Synopfis, Salix, alba, vulgaris, the
common white Willow. Hæc omnium nobis cognita-
rum maxima eft, et in fatis craffam et proceram Ar-
borem adolefcit.

It is called in thefe parts, by the common people,
the willow, and fometimes the Dutch willow; but,
if it be of a foreign extraction, it hath been fo long
naturalized to this climate, that it thrives as well
in it as if it was in its original foil. It is eafily diftin-
guifhed by the notable bitternefs and the free running
of its bark, which may be readily feparated from it
all the fummer months whilft the fap is up. I took
it from the fhoots of three or four years growth, that
fprung from Pollard trees, the diameters of which
fhoots,

123

[199]

shoots, at their biggest end, were from one to four or five inches: it is possible, and indeed not improbable, that this cortex, taken from larger or older shoots, or from the trunk of the tree itself, may be stronger; but I have not had time nor opportunities to make the experiments, which ought to be made upon it. The bark, I had, was gathered in the northern parts of Oxfordshire, which are chiefly of dry and gravelly nature, affording few moist or moory places for this tree to grow in; and therefore, I suspect that its bark is not so good here as in some other parts of the king-dom. Few vegetables are equal in every place; all have their peculiar soils, where they arrive to a greater perfection than in any other place: the best and strongest Mustard-seed is gathered in the county of Durham; the finest Saffron-Flowers are produced in some particular spots of Essex and Cambridgeshire; the best Cyder-apples grow in Herefordshire, De-vonshire and the adjacent counties; the roots of Valerian are esteemed most medicinal, which are dug up in Oxfordshire and Glocestershire: And there-fore why may not the Cortex Salignus, or Cortex Anglicanus, have its favourite soil, where it may flo-rish most, and attain to its highest perfection? It is very probable that it hath; and perhaps it may be in the fens of Lincolnshire, Cambridgeshire, Essex, Kent, or some such like situations; and, though the bark, which grew in the county of Oxford, may seem in some particular cases to be a little inferior to the quinquina, yet, in other places, it may equal, if not exceed it.

The powders made from this bark are at first of a light brown, tinged with a dusky yellow, and the longer they are kept, the more they incline to a

cinnamon

[200]

cinnamon or lateritious colour, which I believe is the cafe with the Peruvian bark and powders.

I have no other motives for publishing this valuable fpecific, than that it may have a fair and full trial in all its variety of circumftances and fituations, and that the world may reap the benefits accruing from it. For thefe purpofes I have given this long and minute account of it, and which I would not have troubled your Lordfhip with, was I not fully perfuaded of the wonderful efficacy of this Cortex Salignus in agues and intermitting cafes, and did I not think, that this perfuafion was fufficiently fupported by the manifold experience, which I have had of it.

I am, my Lord,

with the profoundeft fubmiffion and refpect,

Chipping-Norton,   your Lordfhip's moft obedient
Oxfordfhire,
April 25, 1763.   humble Servant

Edward Stone.

Note: "Edmund Stone" in salutation, "Edward Stone" at signature.

125

Chapter 6

Opioid peptides and pain

Ashley Grossman

There are many species of poppy, but from the fruit of only one of them, *papaver somniferum*, can opiate alkaloids be extracted. However, these compounds are extraordinarily potent analgesics and for millennia they have been used as sedatives and euphoriants. In spite of this, only relatively recently has it been realised that the opiates are counterparts of an endogenous series of opioid compounds, and only twelve years ago were the first opioid peptides sequenced. It is now clear that the endogenous opioids are of fundamental importance in biological function, although their precise role remains far from obvious. Many neuropeptides have been identified and studied in the mammalian nervous system over the last decade, but it is the opioid receptor, almost uniquely, which has any pharmacological "history" prior to the present century.

Historical perspective

Other chapters in this volume have concentrated on analgesics and soporifics in early civilisations, such as the Greek and Roman, and opiates were certainly known and used over two thousand years ago. However, regular use of opium is first recorded in the Far East. Early records are scanty, but both opium eating and smoking appear to have been in frequent use for several centuries. In India, opium eating was particularly popular and was used therapeutically for several

127

conditions, including dysentery and diarrhoea. This latter use is now supported by the extensive pharmacological data on the effects of opiates on gastrointestinal motility, and may be the endogenous equivalent of loperamide for "travellers' diarrhoea". In addition, in Rajputana Province opium was used as a drink "of reconciliation and ordinary greeting". An interesting observation at that time was that "its moderate use may be and is indulged in for years without producing any decided or appreciable ill effects, except weakening the reproductive powers" (Vincent Richards, quoted by Browne[1]). The interaction of endogenous opioids with reproduction is now the object of considerable study (see below).

Opium smoking was more common in China, or where Chinese was the dominant culture, and is recorded as starting around the 17th century, being boosted by foreign opium in the 18th century. As far as can be ascertained, opium smoking was used as a mild stimulant, and in many individuals appears to have been a normal part of social intercourse, as is alcohol or tobacco in our society.

Nevertheless, there is no doubt that a considerable extension of the habit was induced by British traders in the early 19th century. These traders saw the opium market as a means of importing Chinese goods to Europe at very little cost. Not surprisingly, the Chinese authorities took considerable exception to this attitude, but in a far from glorious episode of British history the Opium Wars (1837–1841) clearly established the hegemony of the British opium trade (Figure 1). Such was the success of this economic exploitation that by 1906 it was estimated that 27% of adult males in China smoked opium.

To be fair, it was far from evident to the British at that time that opium was a particularly heinous substance associated with deleterious consequences. Tincture of laudanum was in use in polite circles in London as a mild soporific, and the literati were certainly extensively dabbling in the use of opiates. The influence of opium on Coleridge is well known, and in his Hampstead garden in 1819 John Keats wrote in *Ode to a Nightingale*:

> My heart aches, and a drowsy numbness pains
> My sense, as though of hemlock I had drunk,
> Or emptied some dull opiate to the drains
> One minute past, and lethe-wards had sunk.

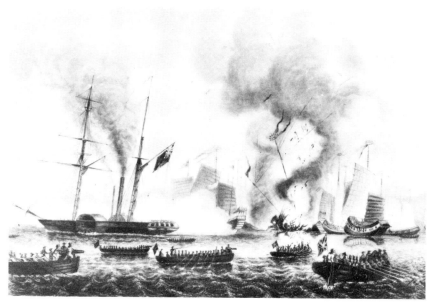

Figure 1 The steamboat "Nemesis" of the East India Company and its associated boats attacking Chinese war junks, in an episode from the Anglo-Chinese Opium Wars (7 January, 1841). (Courtesy of BBC Hulton Picture Library)

It is unlikely that Keats would have written this unless he could assume that his audience, albeit a cultivated and select group, had some acquaintance with the effects of opiates. Similarly, Thomas de Quincey, author of *Confessions of an Opium Eater*, wrote:

> Thou hast the keys of Paradise, oh just,
> Subtle, and mighty opium!

Even Charles Kingsley, not otherwise noted for his involvement in drug trafficking, could complain about the misuse of holy writ as "a Constable's handbook — an opium dose for keeping beasts of burden patient while they are being overloaded". The darker side of opiate use was also manifest in London, where opium-dens, particularly in the Chinese quarter of Limehouse, were a constant feature of Victorian life, and are often cited in contemporaneous novels and detective fiction (Figure 2). Nevertheless, it appeared to be generally considered that opiates were an acceptable "recreational drug", a mild stimulant in low doses but soporific at higher doses, and even in 1929 Browne[1] could write: "Opium smoking (when carried to excess) becomes an inveterate habit, chiefly in individuals of weak will power who would just as easily become the victims of intoxicating drinks, and who are practically moral imbeciles, often addicted also to other forms of depravity." Not until the mid-20th century, and even more recently in the United Kingdom, has widespread opiate-dependence been considered a significant social evil.

Scientific study of the opiates progressed but little in the early decades of this century, although the basic pharmacology of morphine and dihydromorphine (or heroin) was described. However, as anatomical concepts of localisation of brain function were followed by neurochemical advances, including the studies of Barger and Dale[2]

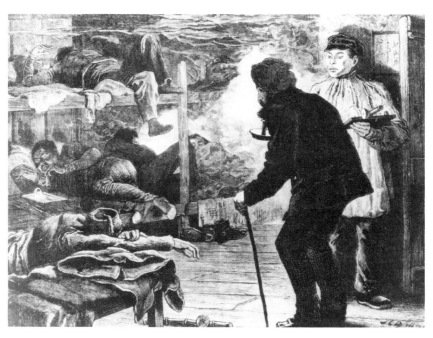

Figure 2 Engraving of an opium-den in London's East End (1880). (Courtesy of BBC Hulton Picture Library)

and Von Euler[3] on neurotransmitters, it generally became realised that specific effects of drugs could best be explained by combination with specific structures or receptors. Furthermore, these receptors were likely to possess their own endogenous ligands. The isolation of opiate receptors proved particularly difficult, as non–specific binding of the radioactively-labelled ligands interfered with the detection of specific binding sites. However, in 1973 two groups identified specific opiate binding in mammalian brain, and the quest for the endogenous ligands for these receptors proceeded at full pace.

Endogenous opioid peptides

In 1975, Hans Kosterlitz and his co-workers[4] at the Unit for Research on Addictive Drugs in Aberdeen were the first to identify and se-quence endogenous opioid peptides, the enkephalins, from porcine brain. These two pentapeptides, methionine-enkephalin and leucine enkephalin, are potent opioid agonists in conventional bioassays, and are highly analgesic when administered to various species intra-cerebroventricularly; they are also rapidly degraded both *in vivo* and *in vitro* by tissue enkephalinase enzymes. Prior to their discovery C. H. Li[5] in San Francisco had identified a novel peptide from the pituitary of the camel, which he named β-lipotrophin (β-LPH), as it had (very slight) lipolytic activity. In 1977, both his group and workers at the National Institute for Medical Research in Mill Hill, London[6], demonstrated that a cleavage product of β-LPH was highly active in opiate bioassays. This peptide consisted of 31 amino-acids and was christened "β-endorphin", as it was envisaged as "endogenous mor-phine". β-endorphin is more resistant to enzyme degradation than the enkephalins, but when it is further cleaved to α-endorphin or γ-endorphin, or when it is acetylated, it loses its opiate activity. Although the first five amino-acids of β-endorphin are identical to those in methionine-enkephalin and are probably responsible for its opiate activity, there is now overwhelming evidence that the enkephalins and endorphins are derived from separate precursors. Indeed, more recently a third family of opioids has been described, the dynorphins, which are amongst the most potent (Greek *dynos* = power) opioids known and tend to have leucine-enkephalin at their

131

active terminus. Thus, three families of opioids are known to exist in the mammalian nervous system.

Opiate receptors

Early pharmacological studies clearly demonstrated that various opiate alkaloids behaved differently in different models, and the concept gradually developed that opiate receptors may be heterogeneous. Thus, morphine was thought to act at its specific μ-receptor, while the principal actions of drugs related to ethylketocyclazocine were considered to be mediated by ϰ-receptors. Both drugs could induce tolerance and dependence in animal models, but there was no cross-tolerance between these two classes of drugs. A third receptor, the σ-receptor, was defined in terms of sensitivity to the prototypal agonist N–allynormetazocine, but it remains uncertain whether this is a true opiate receptor. The use of *in vitro* bioassays and receptor-binding assays, as well as the discovery of the endogenous opioids, has further extended the number of opiate receptors, adding δ-receptors (particularly sensitive to the enkephalin pentapeptides) and possibly ε-receptors (highly sensitive to β-endorphin, but not to morphine).

As each receptor sub-type has its own differential distribution, and as each opioid precursor and its variants of processing are also concentrated in different central nervous system locations, there is considerable complexity in the overall pattern of opioid pathways within the nervous system. Nevertheless, certain basic features are beginning to appear in the structure of the endogenous opioid system. In the brain, the enkephalins are mostly associated with small inhibitory interneurons concentrated in the basal ganglia, limbic system, hypothalamus, and brain stem: they probably act at δ-receptors. Neurons synthesising β-endorphin are almost wholly centred on the arcuate nucleus in the hypothalamus, but these send long axonal processes to many brain regions, including the periaqueductal gray (PAG) in the midbrain. A few β-endorphin-containing cells may also be found in the nucleus tractus solitarius (NTS) in the brain stem. The β-endorphin network is also inhibitory, at μ-receptors and ε-receptors, but may act at longer distances and for longer durations, that is, it may function as a neuromodulator rather than a neurotransmitter system. The dynorphins are located throughout the brain, but are prominent in the substantia gelatinosa of the spinal cord (where the enkephalins may also be found). They appear preferentially to activate $\varkappa$-receptors.

Outside the CNS, opioids may also be found in other organs, particularly the gut and the sympathetic nervous system. Enkephalins are greatly concentrated in the adrenal medulla, where they are co-stored and co-released with adrenaline. Processing of the enkephalin precursor in this site may be incomplete, generating fragments such as "adrenorphin", which may activate μ- or $\varkappa$-receptors. Pro-opiomelanocortin in the anterior pituitary is partially cleaved to produce very low circulating concentrations of β-endorphin; met-enkephalin also circulates in man, but no dynorphin is detectable in human plasma.

Pain and acupuncture

There is no doubt that, in the rat, various forms of analgesia can be associated with activation of endogenous opioid pathways. A large number of studies have clearly shown that stress-induced analgesia is opioid-dependent, while stimulation of the PAG releases central β-endorphin which increases pain tolerance at μ- or ε-receptors. Studies in man are more difficult to organise and assess, but data from the use of naloxone and the measurement of opioids in the cerebro-spinal fluid (CSF) have indicated that endogenous opioid analgesia can be obtained under certain circumstances. This includes the "placebo effect", e. g., the demonstration of analgesia induced by an inactive substance which is believed to be active, but in both rat and man the parameters necessary to demonstrate an effect of endogenous opioids are very precise. It would appear that the pathways involved are complex and involve multiple transmitters in addition to the opioids.

Can these pathways be reliably and regularly activated in man? There is good evidence that certain forms of acupuncture may increase central opioids, but the situations in which this is clinically useful are unclear. Using electroacupuncture (EAP), Dr Wen in collaboration with Dr Clement-Jones[7] showed that high-frequency EAP applied to the ear attenuated the symptoms of heroin-withdrawal by increasing the central release of met-enkephalin; conversely, low-frequency body EAP induces a rise in CSF β-endorphin, probably originating in the PAG, which is associated with analgesia. It seems that we are beginning to obtain evidence in favour of the "gate theory of pain" of Melzack and Wall[8], in which small-diameter pain fibres enter the spinal cord and are then subject to modulation of their input. These fibres access the cord in the substantia gelatinosa, where local inter-neurons containing enkephalins or dynorphins, or long descending pathways controlled by β-endorphin, may "gate out" pain-related impulses. Unfortunately, our ability to selectively activate these pathways remains very limited, and EAP has not proved as useful as was originally hoped. Transcutaneous neural stimulation may also activate these opioid networks, although in practice its efficiency is not contigent upon whether opioids are indeed involved.

As discussed elsewhere in this volume, hypnosis appears to involve higher cortical centres; hypnosis-induced analgesia may decrease pain perception, but there is evidence that this does not involve any opioid mediation.

Opioids: cancer, psychiatry, stress ...

Endogenous opioids have also been implicated in a wide range of other pathophysiological states, but not all of these suggested roles are well buttressed with facts. Some malignancies, particularly carcinoids and small-cell bronchial tumours, may ectopically secrete opioid peptides, and it has been suggested that certain of the psychiatric manifestations of malignant disease may be secondary to these compounds. However, as these peptides have only very limited access to the central nervous system, it is difficult to ascribe to them a major role in mental dysfunction. The opioids have also generated a great deal of enthusiasm in psychiatry, with putative roles as both endogenous neuroleptics and psychotogenic agents being postulated; this has been tempered by the almost uniform finding of minimal or no effect of opioid agonists and antagonists on psychiatric disease in randomised double-blind trials.

In neuroendocrinology, the results look a little more sanguine. It has long been recognised that opiate alkaloids interfere with gonadal function, inducing amenorrhoea in women, impotence in men, and infertility in both. It has now been clearly demonstrated[9] that an endogenous opioid (probably hypothalamic β-endorphin) mediates the inhibition of gonadotrophin secretion seen in women with hyperprolactinaemia (Figure 3). As this is a relatively common condition and lowering of serum prolactin is not always readily achieved, it will be important to see whether long-term opiate blockade will restore regular menstrual cycles in women with hyperprolactinaemic amenorrhoea.

During exercise serum prolactin and growth hormone may rise to considerable levels, and in professional athletes these changes

PLASMA LH & FSH RESPONSE TO NALOXONE IN A PATIENT WITH HYPERPROLACTINAEMIA

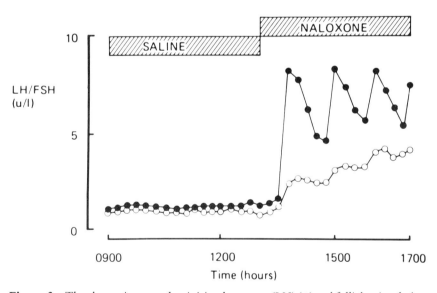

Figure 3 The change in serum luteinising hormone (LH) (●) and follicle stimulating hormone (FSH) (○) in a patient with hyperprolactinaemia who was infused with saline followed by high-dose intravenous naloxone. Note that the low levels of the gonadotrophins increase and become normally pulsatile following the opiate antagonist. (Reproduced from Grossman and colleagues[3], with the permission of the authors and publishers)

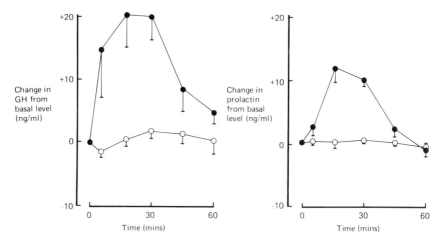

Figure 4   The change in mean (± standard error of mean) serum prolactin and growth hormone (GH) in eight professional athletes undergoing acute severe exercise on a bicycle, with (○) and without (●) an intravenous infusion of high-dose naloxone. Note that the rise in hormones in these subjects is blocked by the naloxone. (Reproduced from Moretti and co-workers[4], with the permission of the authors and publishers)

can be blocked by naloxone[10] (Figure 4). As naloxone does not affect these changes in normal subjects undergoing acute physical exercise, this suggests that it is the process of training as such that activates the endogenous opioid system. However, it should be remembered that circulating opioids do not have ready access to the central nervous system, so exercise-induced changes in their levels cannot be responsible for the "jogger's high" (if it exists).

Finally, recent studies from our department have demonstrated the involvement of endogenous opioids in cardiovascular regulation: any form of stress which activates the sympathetic nervous system and adrenal medulla also increases opioid tone, which acts to damp down or attenuate the sympathoadrenal response. We have therefore suggested that the opioids operate as a major counter-regulatory system to the body's response to stress, preventing excessive activation of sympathetic pathways and modulating their responsiveness (Figures 5 and 6). It is possible that this counter-regulatory system may itself become overactive in shock states and account for the

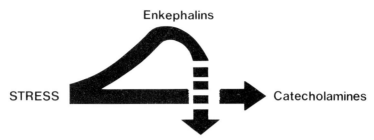

Figure 5 Diagrammatic representation of the role of stress in increasing sympathetic activation, and at the same time releasing an opioid (? enkephalin) brake to attenuate this responsiveness

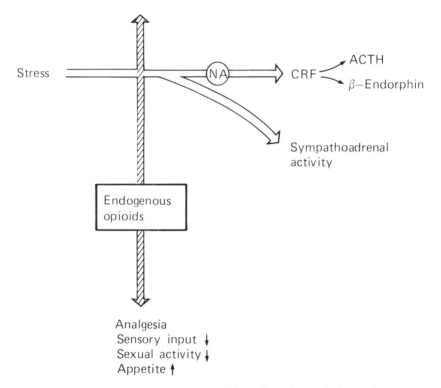

Figure 6 Diagrammatic representation of the effect of stress in increasing various stress axes, including corticotrophin releasing factor (CRF) and adrenocorticotrophin (ACTH), and the sympathetic nervous system. There is evidence that endogenous opioids tonically inhibit a noradrenaline (NA) pathway controlling CRF, phasically attenuate sympathetic responses, and also mediate behavioural changes.

therapeutic benefits of naloxone seen in some patients in intensive care units.

Where next?

While our biochemical and physiological understanding of the effects of opiate alkaloids is relatively advanced, this has made little impact on clinical practice. The opioids are no more effective than the alkaloids in inducing analgesia, and indeed tend to be shorter-acting and have poorer penetration of the brain. Respiratory depression, and phenomena of dependence and tolerance remain equally problematic. Nevertheless, as our understanding of pain and its receptors increases, it seems likely that the delivery of more effective pain relief cannot be too far away. The opiate ϰ-receptors, in addition to μ-receptors, appear to be involved in analgesia, and "designer drugs" for these receptors may have certain advantages over conventional μ-agonists such as morphine or mixed agonist-antagonists such as pentazocine. In addition, preliminary attempts at inducing analgesia by blocking enzyme degradation of endogenous opioids are underway.

However, in the long term it may well be that the opiates will lead the way to a fuller comprehension of stress in all its manifestations, including the apparent need for many susceptible individuals to become dependent on opiates. We have moved a long way from the tincture of laudanum to world-wide opiate abuse and dependence, but the unravelling of stress and the opiate receptor appears near at hand.

Acknowledgement

I am most grateful to Miss Alison Platts for secretarial assistance.

References

1. Browne, F. (1929). Opium. In *Encyclopaedia Britannica*, 14th edn, pp 809–12. London: Encyclopaedia Britannica Ltd
2. Barger, G. and Dale, H. H. (1910). Chemical structure and sympathomimetic action of amines. *J. Physiol.*, **41**, 19–59
3. Von Euler, U. S. (1956). *Noradrenaline*. Springfield, Illinois: Charles C. Thomas

4. Hughes, J., Smith, T. W., Kosterlitz, H. W., Fothergill, L. A., Morgan, B. A. and Morris, H. R. (1975). Identification of two related pentapeptides from the brain with potent opiate agonist activity. *Nature*, **258**, 577–9

5. Li, C. H. (1964). Lipotropin, a new active peptide from pituitary glands. *Nature*, **201**, 924–5

6. Bradbury, A. F., Smyth, D. G., Snell, C. R., Birdsall, N. J. M. and Hulme, E. C. (1976). C fragment of lipotropin has a high affinity for brain opiate receptors. *Nature*, **260**, 793–5

7. Clement-Jones, V., McLoughlin, L., Lowry, P. J., Besser, G. M., Rees, L. H. and Wen, H. L. (1979). Acupuncture in heroin addicts: changes in met-enkephalin and β-endorphin in blood and cerebrospinal fluid. *Lancet*, **ii**, 380–3

8. Melzack, R. and Wall, P. D. (1965). Pain mechanisms: a new theory. *Science*, **150**, 971–9

9. Grossman, A., Moult, P. J. A., McIntyre, H., Evans, J., Silverstone, T., Rees, L. H. and Besser, G. M. (1982). Opiate mediation of amenorrhoea in hyperprolactinaemia and in weight-loss related amenorrhoea. *Clin. Endocrinol.*, **17**, 379–88

10. Moretti, C., Fabbri, A., Gnessi, L., Cappa, M., Calzolari, A., Grossman, A. and Besser, G. M. (1983). Naloxone inhibits exercise-induced release of PRL and GH in athletes. *Clin. Endocrinol.*, **18**, 135–8

Reviews

1. Watson, S. J., Akil, H., Richard, C. W. and Barchas, J. D. (1978). Evidence for two separate opiate peptide neuronal systems. *Nature*, **275**, 226–8

2. Morley, J. E. (1981). The endocrinology of the opiates and opioid peptides. *Metabolism*, **30**, 195–209

3. Grossman, A. (1983). Brain opiates and neuroendocrine function. In Scanlon, M. F. (ed.) *Clinics in Endocrinology and Metabolism*, Vol. 12 (3) "Neuroendocrinology", pp 725–46. Eastbourne: W. B. Saunders & Co.

4. Skrabanek, P. (1984). Acupuncture and the age of unreason. *Lancet*, **1**, 1169–71

5. MacKay, A. V. P. (1985). Neuropeptides and psychiatry. In Granville-Grossman, K. (ed.) *Recent Advances in Clinical Psychiatry*, Vol. 5, pp 179–200. Edinburgh: Churchill Livingstone

6. Grossman, A., Clement-Jones, V. and Besser, G. M. (1985). Clinical implications of endogenous opioid peptides. In Müller, E. E., MacLeod, R. M. and Frohman, L. A. (eds) *Neuroendocrine Perspectives*, Vol. 4, pp 243–94. Amsterdam: Elsevier

7. Bouloux, P. M. G. (1987). Cardiovascular responses to stress: the role of opioid peptides. In Grossman, A. (ed.) *Baillière's Clinical Endocrinology and Metabolism — International Practice and Research. The Neuroendocrinology of Stress*. London: Harcourt Brace. (In press)

Chapter 7

The pain of psychosis

Malcolm P. I. Weller

A historical survey of care

The pain of psychosis is psychological, indeed the capacity to feel physical pain seems to be blunted. The possible biochemical reasons for this are discussed later in this chapter. Paradoxically, this relative indifference to discomfort, cold and hunger contributes to the destitution and neglect that may readily befall psychotic patients not having hospital care, who may easily circulate between acute psychiatric admissions, destitution and imprisonment. This problem is perennial and the history of British psychiatry is replete with themes that vividly reflect contemporary problems.

In Saxon times families had to care for their mentally disordered relatives, the nearest male relative bearing the responsibility for protecting the public. The burden of responsibility was decided initially by an official — the Chancellor — and later by jury and imposed by the Chancellor. The first statutes dealing with these matters were passed in the reign of Edward II and in Scotland at the beginning of the 14th century.

In the 15th century an opportunity was provided for the mentally disturbed to be cared for either at home or under ecclesiastical auspices. At the same time, belief in witches and demons convulsed Europe under the pernicious influence of the *Malleus Maleficarum* (*The Witch Hammer*). This work, written by two misogynist, Dominican,

141

German theologians — Johann Sprenger and Heinrich Krämer, who ironically styled themselves "dogs of the Lord" (*canes Dominii*) — was published in 1487 and given papal approval by Innocent VIII. Even though it now seems absurd, it led to the torture and execution of the mentally ill, under the pretext of religion, advocating that, after protestations of mercy by all connected with the examination, the Judge should finally come in and "promise that he will be merciful, with the mental reservation that he means he will be merciful to himself or the State …"[1].

It was dangerous in the extreme to speak out against this abuse but the forces of the Reformation, as expressed by such men as Erasmus, Sir Thomas Moore and Luther, were slowly undermining the established order and in 1563 Johann Weyer, a German physician writing under the patronage and protection of Duke William of Jülich, Berg and Cleves, published the results of his study of witchcraft trials, in his important critique, *Delusions of Witches*.

The belief in demonology never again caused the same savage consequences but the aura and stigmatisation linger. In 1922 the Reverend Hugh W. White, a doctor of divinity, published a work, *Demonism Verified and Analysed*, which purported to show that mental illness exemplified demonic forces. The belief remains entrenched; the film *The Exorcist* became an unprecedented commercial success and ushered in successors with a similar theme, such as the *Omen* series, *Halloween*, *Poltergeist* and *Zombie Lake*. All of these helped to sustain an interest in the occult and reinforced prejudices about the Satanic origins of abnormal mental states. One of my patients died in *status epilepticus* after his vicar, with whom he was living, induced him to abandon his anti–epileptic medication in favour of prayer.

The broad sweep of contemporary legislation takes a discernible origin from the Vagrancy Act 1714, which provided an opportunity whereby two or more Justices of the Peace could ensure the safe keeping of someone who was dangerously insane. This could continue only whilst the person was mad but there was no provision for medical attention. The 1714 Act was replaced in 1743 by the Justices Commitment Act, when cure was first mentioned; again the possibility of a friend or relative providing protection was emphasised as an alternative to institutional care. When those who were detained because of madness were released, parishes were relieved of the financial burden.

Humane and liberal treatment of the mentally ill in France, impelled particularly by Phillipe Pinel (1754–1826) and Jean Esquirol (1772–1840), had an influence on English thought. Pinel took the revolutionary step of unchaining his patients at Bicêtre Hospital in 1793. Esquirol exerted a profound influence on the thought of his time, advocating the treatment of the criminally insane and distinguishing them from other prisoners. Moral treatment, a combination of humanitarianism and Christianity, was emphasised by William Tuke (1732–1822), a prosperous Quaker tea merchant who built the Retreat at York in 1792 as an alternative to the York Asylum. His methods can be seen as forerunners of modern behavioural techniques. The Retreat was intended to be used exclusively by Quakers and Tuke was thought imprudent to design it for what was imagined to be an excessive capacity of 30, but numbers rose persistently and reached 71 in 1840.

Prison: the King's pleasure

James Hatfield's attempt on the life of George III was a seminal event in medico-legal history. Hatfield was considered sane and fit to stand trial by the King's brother, who examined him directly after the event; but his counsel, Erskine, was able to persuade the court that his client was suffering from paranoid delusions. Although he was thereby acquitted of treason, by virtue of his madness, he was not released, as had been the practice hitherto, but was transferred to Newgate prison. The Criminal Lunatics Act of 1800 was rushed through Parliament, with retrospective effect to accommodate this disposal. It ordered that dangerous lunatics should be detained "in strict custody" during the King's pleasure. Magistrates were dissatisfied that lunatics were deprived of their freedom whether or not their pleas were upheld. They were also dissatisfied "to confine such persons in a common Goal, (which) is equally destructive of the recovery of the insane and of the comfort of the other prisoners"[2]. Both these problems remain with us today. Secure custody was difficult to realise then, as it is to some extent even now. Hatfield was subsequently transferred to Bethlem Hospital and during a fracas killed a patient there.

143

In 1807 the Select Committee came to the conclusion, still relevant today, that many of the people who were in prison should in fact be in hospital. The County Asylums Act was passed in 1808; it incorporated the 1744 and 1800 Acts and dealt with the detention of both pauper lunatics and those who were able to pay.

Scandal and change

A number of scandals involving financial mismanagement and in-adequacies of care were exposed in the asylums and these impelled legislative changes. Amongst the most notorious was the case of William Norris, who was confined at Bethlem. It was described by Edward Wakefield, who was largely responsible for the 1815 Parliamentary Select Committee to which Tuke, amongst others, gave evidence. "It was impossible for him to advance from the wall … on account of the shortness of his chains, which were only twelve inches long. It was, I conceive, equally out of his power to repose in any other position than on his back, the projections which on each side of his waist bar enclosed his arms, rendering it impossible for him to lie on his side …" Wakefield also noted that there were many who were chained, covered only by blankets, "their nakedness and their mode of confinement gave this room the appearance of a dog kennel."

Scandals continued and in 1829 it was found that patients had been kept in wooden cages covered with straw over the weekends. Sufficient food was put in for them to survive this period. When it ended they were taken out and cleansed of accumulated faeces with a mop.

In 1835 a House of Lords Select Committee complained again, once more with contemporary relevance, that it was difficult to transfer the mentally ill from prison because alternative facilities were often full. In the same year, representatives of Hanwell Asylum wrote to the Home Secretary pointing out that they did not really have secure facilities. This was a particular source of difficulty, not only for the protection of the public and the insane, but also because fines of £2–10 were imposed upon the custodians when patients absconded. In the purchasing power of the day this was a very considerable sum, which moreover was soon raised to £20.

Expansion of the asylums

The Lunacy Act of 1845, largely framed by Lord Shaftesbury, established a Board of Commissioners empowered to license metropolitan institutions. Each was required to keep appropriate records and the Commissioners produced three yearly reports; magistrates continued to license provincial institutions. All of the legislation to this time had led to detention of mentally ill people in secure facilities for indeterminate periods and it was the Commissioners' duty to visit all the insane, whether or not they were in asylums.

The confidence of Tuke that demand would fill the Retreat could already be demonstrated. A national survey by the Commissioners drew attention to the extent of the demand for asylum whereby "it has been found necessary to enlarge every asylum of that sort that has hitherto been erected ... and some of them several times." This pressure continued to be felt although at least £10 million in capital was expended on the creation of the asylums and £1½ million was expended on their annual upkeep.

Review of detention

The Lunacy Act 1845 provided for the review of patients in a way which can be seen as the forerunner of the Mental Health Review Tribunal. This Act placed a statutory obligation on counties and boroughs to provide, within three years, adequate asylum provision for pauper lunatics. The Commissioners in Lunacy had been struck by the accumulation of the chronic cases in these asylums and felt, like many present-day commentators, that alternative provisions should be created "in order to make room for others whose cases had not yet become hopeless. If some plan of this sort be not adopted the Asylums admitting paupers will necessarily continue full of incurable patients ... and the skill and labour of the physician will thus be wasted upon improper objects."[3]

The Mental Health Act 1959

There was a final 1889 Lunacy Act, making at least forty statutes relating to insanity in England and eight in Scotland between then and 1300, before the passing of the Mental Treatment Act 1930 in which voluntary admissions were first countenanced, the voluntary patients

145

signing a form requesting admission. This formality was discarded in the 1959 Mental Health Act, the main emphasis of which was to encourage voluntary admission, described as *informal*. The Act also placed emphasis on local authorities to provide residential and training centres for patients whose condition did not call for full hospital care, but who nevertheless needed some form of rehabilitation, shelter or supervision. This was a purposeful time when the adverse effects of confinement and understimulation were beginning to be recognised, and followed the introduction of chlorpromazine into this country in 1955, which had such a profound effect on treatment practice. The slow evolution and failures of community care can be largely attributed to the failure of local authorities to respond adequately to the provisos in the 1959 Mental Health Act.

There had been a fear that compulsion would be used inappropriately. A House of Commons Select Committee exhaustively examined the operation of the law in 1877 and concluded that they were unable to identify a single case of inappropriate detention. In 1890, Chambers Encyclopaedia estimated that 40% of patients treated in asylums recovered but that many relapsed "from which, however, they often recover again, just as people have relapses in rheumatism and bronchitis". The recovery rate was estimated at 70% if "there was no organic brain disease nor very advanced senility". The death rate was estimated to be about five times that of the general population and the Commissioners' reports, published in the *Journal of Mental Health*, identified syphylis as the principal cause of death, with tuberculosis not far behind, although a far-sighted comment of the time was that "insanity is in fact a disease of the brain, from which people die as from other diseases".

A history of mistakes

In many ways the situation was commendable but pessimism about the patients' ability to cope and their limited potential for rehabilitation led to a custodial role for the psychiatric hospitals. Patients were deprived of even small tokens of individual preferences and were sometimes not allowed to own a comb or toothbrush. This unsatisfactory, nihilistic and antitherapeutic ambience was identified and emphasis gradually placed on individual choice and stimulation as essential components of active rehabilitation programmes[4]. This work is still cited as though sociologists or social workers were the exclusive critics of earlier psychiatric practice, and as though no notice had been taken of the message that some of the apparent features of the psychiatric diseases (mostly schizophrenia) were exacerbated by deficiencies in the system of care and the level of staffing.

Indeed, the boot is much more on the other foot and the "liberal", *laissez faire* policies that dominate local authority hostels frequently lead to the rapid undermining of the benefits obtained in careful, prolonged behaviour programmes which have been devised and run in hospital settings. This is a regrettable situation that I repeatedly witness in my role as consultant to a supra-district intensive rehabilitation ward[5].

The initial impetus for psychiatric hospital closures in the UK originated in a dubious extrapolation of hospital discharge figures, which was published in the same year as Goffman's polemic entitled *Asylums*, in a paper by Tooth and Brooke[6] that drew methodological criticisms. This paper, which appeared close in time to two others discussing general hospital closures, predicted that the long-stay population was declining at such a rate that it would be eliminated in about sixteen years. It was thought that replacement would generate a need for 890 long-stay beds per million of the population and an overall figure of 1800 beds per million for all types of care. These predictions were discussed in a subsequent editorial in 1961[7], which stated "All share the Minister of Health's hope that the number of beds in mental hospitals can be safely reduced." (Plus c'est change c'est plus la même chose.) Quite apart from the illogicality of extrapolating an alleged linear trend to extinction, the figures cited by Dr Tooth and Miss Brooke did not seem to justify the linear trend of decline they assumed:

Long-stay patients in hospital on Dec. 31, 1954		112 113
Deaths and discharges	1955	8 163
	1956	7 432
	1957	6 608
	1958	6 249
	1959	5 953

All three papers were partly based on subjective assessments which, as one critical correspondent pointed out, "are still matters of opinion, even when expressed as percentages to the first decimal place"[8]. Nonetheless, even if closures are not to take place at a pace determined by the sustained rate of discharge of long-stay patients, with an inconsequential build-up of "new" long-stay patients, the objective of psychiatric hospital closures is still being actively pursued[9]. One must be anxious that the right policy be found and that it proceed successfully.

The prescient words of Egan[10], discussing the contentious Tooth and Brooke extrapolation of bed reductions, seem apposite: "Areas like Burnley and Oldham would seem tailor-made for a planned investigation into the effects on family life of keeping chronic psychotics and other permanent invalids at home ... It may show that psychotics find hospital treatment outside of their home areas." The American experiences[11,12] of a drift of the mentally ill to the decaying city centres must be compared with the drift of drug addicts, alcoholics and schizophrenics into London[13,14].

Nevertheless, of "such stuff are dreams made of" and the conclusions of Tooth and Brooke[6] struck a responsive chord. The simple extrapolation was stripped of all caveats and incorporated as policy objectives into the *Hospital Plan for England and Wales* by the Minister of Health, who presented his deliberations to Parliament in 1962. The considerable local variations in bed provision at the time were considered artifactual, undesirable or irrelevant and homogeneous national objectives were created for the numbers of psychiatric beds in relation to the population. The only assumption made regarding social provisions was that if these increased over their low level in the preceding period of the study the extrapolated expectations for hospital facilities would prove unduly conservative!

The recent past

In the UK the peak in psychiatric bed occupancy occurred in 1954. It is often asserted that the subsequent decline occurred before the introduction of the phenothiazine antipsychotic drugs (the first of which was chlorpromazine) and represented a shift in psychiatric attitude; however, the figures hardly bear this out.

Around this same time (mid-1950s) regrets were expressed that psychiatric care was not more readily available in a more open and less intimidating way; the complaints voiced then have a depressingly contemporary ring: "… Psychiatric care cannot yet be said to be *readily* available, except for those whose condition demands immediate admission to hospital…" "The problem is complicated by the resistance which many patients show to anything "psychiatric', regarding the out-patient department as the open door to the 'asylum', and any recommendation for psychiatric treatment may provoke hostility and resentment from which the practitioner may retreat." (MacCalman, 1951, cited by Heimler[15])

Economic factors are important determinants of the outcome, both in terms of the provision of sufficient finance for caring arrangements and in terms of the opportunities for gainful employment for those who have suffered mental illness, particularly those with residual symptoms[16]. Regrettably, both these are areas of difficulty. By the same token one is suspicious that "normalisation", that is, leading as normal a life as possible, will come to imply that nothing special need be created. It is ironical that as the old psychiatric hospitals responded to the criticisms that too little was expected of the patients, who it was wrongly imagined were insensitive to expectations, and as initiatives were energetically pursued to commence socially-based treatment schedules (causing the costs, particularly the staffing costs, to rise considerably), it was decided by the North East Thames Region to close Friern and Claybury hospitals — because they were particularly expensive, despite the fact that they were the inheritors of a generation of financial neglect. Even now, after a halving of the psychiatric hospital beds (see Figure 1) psychiatric patients occupy approximately half the total National Health Service beds, whilst attracting a quarter of the National Health Service expenditure.

The North East Thames Regional Health Authority designated provider groups to evaluate the cost of community provisions for the four districts served by Friern Hospital, to replace the hospital. Some £20 million was projected, compared to the existing hospital budget, including works, of £14 million. The Region then specified a total budget allocation, for this priority service, of £9 million[17]. These are

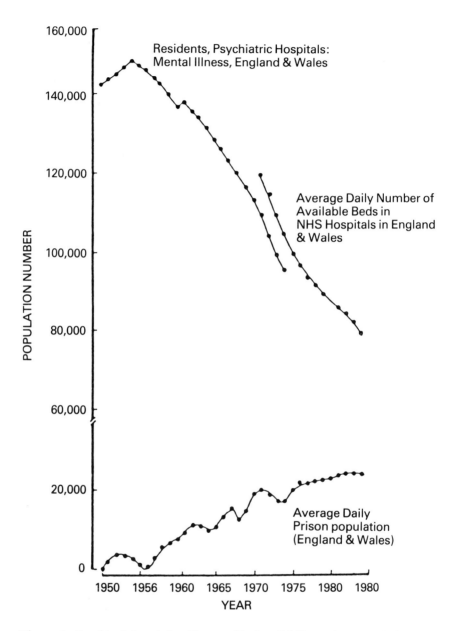

Figure 1 Psychiatric hospital residents and bed availability and average daily prison population in England and Wales since 1950

small sums compared with the £17 billion backlog of NHS repairs and maintenance[18], to which Friern hospital makes a modest £6.5 million contribution, at 1984 prices[19].

Any change in practice, particularly shifting the locus of care to a more accessible community base, has to be handled sensitively so that morale can be maintained. The most crucial period, which may last for ten or more years, lies between the initial announcement of hospital closure and new facilities coming on stream. It should be obvious that staff have to have their futures assured when a hospital is nominated for closure — but staff may be left unnecessarily doubtful and uncertain about the future for want of attention to these obvious considerations.

We compared two well supported out-patient groups with long-stay hospitalised patients and found that the in-patient group had a better quality of life on a number of measures; this despite the fact that in one of the hospitalised groups the patients were significantly older than the comparison out-patient group.

Two groups of in-patients, at two different psychiatric hospitals, St Mary's, Stannington, Northumberland ($n = 40$), and Friern, in North London ($n = 23$), were interviewed, together with out-patients from both hospitals ($n = 40$, St Mary's; $n = 16$, Friern); all the out-patients were actively supported by community nurses. The interviews were conducted according to a prepared schedule that had been piloted, modified and discussed with the nurses prior to use. The nurses, including community psychiatric nurses, held a variety of views on the intended transition to community care.

The Friern in-patients were significantly older than the out-patients ($p < 0.001$) (in-patients: range 37–73, mean 56.5, SD 11.2; out-patients: range 20–64, mean 40.9, SD 13.77) but were carefully matched for age and sex in the St Mary's groups (in-patients: range 23–77, mean 51.3, SD 15.14; out-patients: range 24–73, mean 50.4, SD 13.86).

In all we enquired into twenty indicators of quality of life. Hospitalised patients were significantly advantaged (Mann-Whitney, two tailed probabilities) in terms of attending social gatherings ($p < 0.05$ both groups), going to places of entertainment ($p < 0.001$, St Mary's), the number of meals per week ($p < 0.001$, Friern), the number of hot meals ($p < 0.001$ both groups), and the number of baths per week ($p < 0.005$, St Mary's). As might be expected, the in-patients were also advantaged in the amount of time they spent in rehabilitation programmes ($p < 0.001$, St Mary's), and in passive amusements ($p < 0.05$ St Mary's; $p < 0.05$ Friern watching TV; $p < 0.005$ listening to the radio at St Mary's). However, if contacts with nursing, medical and paramedical staff are disregarded, the Friern in-patients enjoyed less company ($p < 0.01$), which might reflect their advanced age, and they attentively listened less to the radio ($p < 0.005$). In other respects the groups were comparable (Weller, B. G. A., Weller, M. P. I. and Cheyne, A. "Long-term psychiatric patients in the community", *Br. J. Psychiat.* (1987), **151**, 862).

Lessons from America and Italy

We must be careful to preserve what is good in our attempts to do better, and the drive towards community care must not ignore the constructive role that psychiatric hospitals are, however imperfectly, currently performing. The same movement towards hospital closure was highly developed in the USA, where the old hospitals were seen as repositaries of neglected patients for the convenience of staff[20], and efforts were made to replace them, as rapidly as possible, with community mental health centres (CMHC). The enabling legislation, the Community Mental Health Centres Act, was passed by Congress in 1963 and signed into law (Public Law 88-164) by President Kennedy in October of that year. Unfortunately, the initial aspirations for these centres were not fully realised and it quickly became apparent that the centres were incapable of treating and managing the most disturbed patients without a very much greater participation by psychiatrists. Less highly trained staff quickly came to rely on the expertise of psychiatrists to a point where their capacity was excessively stretched[21,22], whilst at the same time the ratio of psychiatrists per CMHC actually diminished, through disenchantment, to less than half between 1970 and 1975 and the proportion of centres with psychiatrists as directors or executive directors fell from 56% in 1973 to 22% in 1977[23].

The Italian experience of closing mental hospitals is portrayed differently by different observers, some being eulogistic, although there are many perturbing features. Whatever the alleged merits of the Italian Mental Health Act of 1978 (Law No. 180), it has been found to be defective; it is currently undergoing revision, with an extension of compulsory powers, an increase in the number of beds for the acutely ill (with opportunities for transfer to medium-stay units if recovery is delayed), and the creation of new long-stay units[24]. The rate of decrease in the number of long-stay patients has actually slowed down since the passage of Law No. 180[25]. This change may therefore be construed as following, rather than leading, the reduction in the long-term population: in a similar fashion to the halving of the UK long-stay patient population, sparing only the most disabled, in advance of the current slogans and enthusiasms.

It has been estimated[26] that only 8.4% of the 4.9 million people using specialised mental health services in the USA in a given year are treated in CMHCs. Inevitably, there was pressure to select patients who could benefit from the new arrangements. A new, and perhaps previously neglected, population was being served by the community health centres, to the detriment of the most severely ill, the chronically ill and the elderly, whilst the traditional services for the most ill were still being conducted in the large psychiatric hospitals[23, 27, 28].

The loss to follow-up of patients out of touch with services is amplified by the fact that in England many have moved away from the districts where they were known[14, 29]. Similar problems have been experienced at Powick Hospital and in Scotland[30], where 40% of those discharged had no contact with after-care services. This figure rose to 75% among discharged first admissions out of 571 "new chronic in-patients" (from many different hospitals) aged between 18 and 64 years and who had spent more than one but less than six years in hospital.

Rural figures belie wide differences and are very much exceeded in the inner London district of Camden, where the point prevalence of schizophrenia is over eight and a half per thousand (Campbell, Harvey and Pantelis, survey given at the G.P. Study Day Symposium, "Psychiatry in Transition: Promoting Community Developments", Friern Hospital, 27th November, 1986). A similarly high figure was recorded in Salford[31], here possibly because of a shifting population as the more enterprising drift away. That schizophrenics both migrate[32-4] and stay put is contradictory, but both tendencies may well operate, and a suitable register could clarify the situation.

Local authority resources

All the planning for community care is focused on the least disabled and envisages selling land and existing buildings and moving National Health Service income to local authorities. One is concerned that the personnel in local authority employ have neither the training nor the skills to provide for the range of psychopathology at present being treated in hospitals.

The confident aspirations of social services to provide a standard of care exceeding that obtainable in psychiatric hospitals is suspect. Training and experience are wanting[35]. Since 1971 social services have had responsibility for community-based services. There has been a steady discharge of long-stay patients at a rate of 2–3000 per annum, amounting to some 70 000 since 1954. Yet only 4000 are residing in local authority provisions and this number is slightly declining, contemporaneously with a reduction in back-up services, such as meals-on-wheels and home helps. Day centres are few and failing to increase in line with guidelines issued in 1975[36]. Much of the work of the social services is discretionary and where statutory obligations towards the mentally ill exist, for example to house the vulnerable homeless, they are subtly evaded[37].

The second Minority Report by Professor R. Pinker, worryingly, yet appropriately, entitled "An alternative view", in the Barclay Committee Report[35] has some sound things to say. Professor Pinker is properly concerned at the continuing dilution of skills and diffusion of effort and argues persuasively for strong professionalism; this involves, amongst other things, clear lines of accountability, a General Social Work Council charged with the maintenance of professional standards, and a planned balance between generic abilities and special-ist skills. This dissenting view from his seventeen colleagues on the Committee and the title of the Report reinforce the concern that the boundaries of social work are too imprecise, as currently constituted, and the statutory obligations insufficient for social workers to be in a strong enough position to achieve a dominant place in community schemes dealing with fragile, vulnerable people. "On the face of it, nothing would seem more obvious than that the profession of psychiatry should take a leading part — if not the leading part — in the development of the mental health service in the community. Beneath the common sense assumption that this is *par excellence* the profession dedicated to the care of the mentally ill, there lies a deeper recognition of the many advances in standards of care that are properly attributable to the work of psychiatrists, from the abolition of locked wards to the spread of Day Hospitals. One might speak also of major contributions to aetiological, epidemiological and therapeutic knowledge ..."[38]

Legislative inadequacies

The existing legislation is inadequate. The obligation to house vulnerable homeless people under the Housing (Homeless Persons) Act 1985 expires if a person should "voluntarily" quit his accommodation and becomes homeless intentionally. Although in other circumstances deluded and hallucinating patients may not be held to have testamentary capacity to enter into binding contracts, they are held to be liable in respect of quitting their accommodation — they subsequently cease to be the responsibility of any authority. This is despite the fact that their mental disability created their priority need. Added to this problem is the extreme difficulty of finding supervised accommodation at all, although they should be provided by entitlement under Part III of the National Assistance Act 1948, which lays out the duties of local authorities "to provide residential accommodation for persons who by reason of age, infirmity or any other circumstances are in need of care and attention which is not otherwise available to them" (subsection 1a). "In the exercise of their said duty a local authority shall have regard to the welfare of all persons for whom accommodation is provided, and in particular to the need for providing accommodation of different descriptions suited to different descriptions of such persons as are mentioned in the last foregoing subsection" (subsection 2). Despite the clear expectations of the Act, there is no local authority known to the author which makes such provision for people under the age of 65.

The hurried passage of the 1983 Mental Health Act created a situation where additional resources were clearly required, but were not forthcoming. Consider, for example, sections 30, 35 and 37, whereby those charged or convicted of offences can be transferred to psychiatric hospitals. The administrative burdens included in these sections require the hospital to deliver the patient to Court at the appointed time, a requirement that, understandably, we have been unable to induce the Court, the police or the probation service to undertake. These reponsibilities and the encouragement of an increased use of Appeal Tribunals, obligatory every six months under the 1983 Act, have generated immense calls on medical time without additional staffing.

A serious flaw is contained in the illusion of local authority responsibility for patients returning home on leave whilst on a treatment order under Section 117 of the Mental Health Act 1983. Indeed, the responsibility that already existed under the National Health Service Act 1977 might have actually been weakened. The local authority is required to provide "after-care services", which are not specified in the Act. In any event Lord Denning (in Southwark L.B.C. *v.* Williams [1971] ch. 734 at p. 743) referred to the principle that "Where an Act creates an obligation, and enforces that obligation in a specified manner, we take it to be a general rule that performance cannot be enforced in any other manner." (See Wyatt *v.* Hillingdon L.B.C., 76 L.G.R. 727.) Section 124 of the Mental Health Act 1983 provides for the Secretary of State to exercise default powers when a local authority fails in its obligations and abrogate to himself such of the functions of the authority as he deems appropriate. It is unlikely that he would ever feel called upon to do so, but the specific provision makes it more unlikely that an individual would be able to enforce section 117.

Local authorities have the ability to provide "centres (including training centres and day centres) or other facilities (including domiciliary facilities) whether in premises managed by the [local authority] or otherwise, for training or occupation of persons suffering from or who have been suffering from mental disorders". This ability, conferred by DHSS Circular No. 19/75[9], is unenforceable, and says no more than the 1977 Act whereby a local authority is *required* to co-operate with the health authority "in order to advance the health and welfare of the people of England and Wales".

One may conclude that in important respects the net effect of the 1983 Act and the DHSS circular has been to weaken the entitlement of patients to local authority provisions, whilst creating a misleading impression that these entitlements have been ensured.

Quantification of requirements

The DHSS (1975) guidelines[39] recommend 4–6 beds in local authority hostels per 100 000 district population, 15–24 beds for long-stay accommodation and 60 day places in day centres. Unfortunately, these figures were not justified by any indication of the means by which they were calculated or the assumptions on which they were based. In effect, therefore, they have no justification. "Whether ideals so loosely expressed and with no solid plan for implementation can properly be described as amounting to a policy is very much open to debate."[40] One cannot readily see that the "caring" landlady scheme, currently so popular with local authorities, represents an appropriate alternative to hospital care, although it is undoubtedly cheaper. The modest targets mentioned are to be "achieved as economic resources allow". One is concerned at the adequacy of these targets, the wide range in the estimates, the lack of rigour in the long-stay accommodation proposals, and the manifest desire to close hospitals hastily in advance of even these inadequate provisions.

The dishevelled self-neglect that typifies the apathetic indifference of the chronic schizophrenic usually leads to social ostracism. There seems to be a penumbra of social acceptability for patients in the close vicinity of psychiatric hospitals, where understanding has built up gradually over the years. This understanding generates an ethos that permeates even to the new residents in the neighbourhood, who seem to absorb the good-natured tolerance. Elsewhere, however, there is manifest hostility to establishing community services, a phenomenon seen in America[41] and in Italy, where day centres have been repeatedly burned down by the angered populace[42].

These concepts have been summarised by Jones[43], who wrote: "The act of discharging a patient is in itself relatively simple. The statement that a patient has been discharged tells us only that he has left hospital, not what the hospital has done for him, in what state he is now, or what the community can do for him. A 'liberal' discharge policy is a kindness to some patients; it could be an instrument of cruelty to

157

others. We should be unwise to place too much reliance on discharge statistics, or to regard them as an index of success."

Failures of community care

There is probably some disturbance of the ability of schizophrenic patients to experience physical pain. They often have severe cigarette burns on their fingers, and seem oblivious to the cold, walking thinly clad in winter without apparent discomfort. "They endure uncomfortable positions, pricks of a needle, injuries, without thinking much about it; burn themselves with their cigar, hurt themselves, tear out the hair of their genitals, let the glaring noonday sun shine in their face for hours, do not chase away flies which settle on their eyelids."[44] This relative indifference to physical discomfort makes schizophrenic patients vulnerable to physical harm and they sometimes sustain horrendous injuries without complaint.

Some disturbance of the opioid systems seems plausible. Psychomimetic effects have been claimed for opiates having partial agonist/antagonist actions, but evidence for abnormalities of β-endorphin in the cerebrospinal fluid of schizophrenics has proved difficult to replicate[45]. Therapeutic claims have been made for the usefulness of the opiate antagonists naloxone and naltrexone[46]; there have also been unsubstantiated claims[47-9] for des-tyr-gamma-endorphin[50]. Van Ree and colleagues[51] have claimed an antipsychotic effect for des-enkephalin-gamma-endorphin in a double-blind placebo controlled trial in thirteen schizophrenic patients.

A more common problem than serious, expectedly painful injuries is that schizophrenic patients, if not very well cared for in community settings, go hungry and sleep in the open with little complaint, when discharged from hospital; they are also sometimes tormented by hallucinations and fearful delusions.

Out of a hundred people interviewed in London in "Crisis at Christmas 1984", a charity providing shelter on Christmas Eve, one in five had positive symptoms of schizophrenia, one in three had definite or probable schizophrenia, and two in five were psychotic at the time of interview (42% of those permitting a mental state examination)[14]. Twelve of the psychotic respondents (13.6%) had never been in contact with psychiatric services, ten (32.3%) were not receiving any benefit entitlement, and twenty-five (80.6%) had been to prison, including one who had been to Broadmoor for attempted murder. More than half of the total interviewed population were either psychotic or had received in-patient psychiatric treatment in the past, including a convicted murderer, and, *pace* the Resource Allocation Working Party (RAWP), over 90% had migrated to London from elsewhere. An impression of this degree of migration is given by the map which forms Figure 2.

Loss of connection from supporting networks is characteristic of mental illness, particularly schizophrenia: 64% of the total destitute population examined on this occasion claimed to have neither friend nor acquaintance, 36% were not receiving any benefits, and 63% had slept rough the previous night — a deterioration from the findings of a similar study conducted the previous year, which nevertheless revealed a similar pattern[52]. It should come as no surprise that community "care", that much vaunted shibboleth, leads to disease and death[53-9] (see also personal communications from the staff at the Camberwell Reception Centre, London, and Dr A. Naftalin, visiting medical officer to Bruce House, London WC2).

As for civil liberties and freedom of choice, only eleven of the six hundred long-stay patients at Friern Hospital are there by compulsion, and many of these are constrained by Court orders. Social services, which currently finance accommodation for the vulnerable, daily express an exquisite concern not to relocate those who do not earnestly wish to leave the hospital, but this is, paradoxically, combined with an enthusiasm to close the hospital entirely. Financial inducements are promised from National Health Service resources to provide care, even though the social services are ill-equipped to give it[35,60], in accordance with a financial formula which seems calculated to wreak disaster, whereby a capitation sum equivalent to the average annual cost in hospital care is given to social services for the long-stay patients they take into their own care. This sum will deplete the hospital, which will be left with the most disturbed patients and continuing fixed costs allowing less money for each patient[19], and no reserve if the discharged patient requires readmission.

Hospitals have a wide range of facilities and amenities — occupational and industrial therapy; music, art, and pottery; psychotherapy, social skills and relaxation classes; specialist diets under the supervision of dieticians; religious services; patient clubs and cafeteria; gymnasiums and remedial gymnasts; specialist services, such as dentistry, chiro-

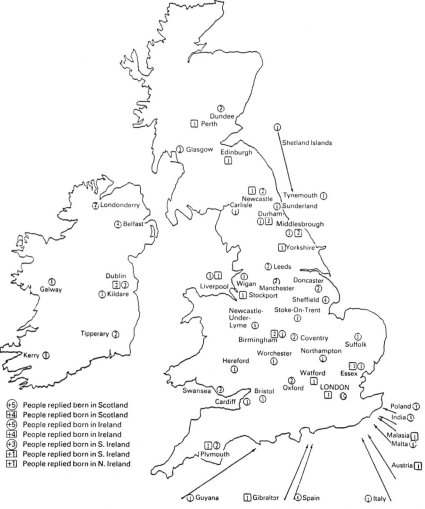

Figure 2 Place of birth of 116 patients interviewed at Christmas in 1985 (□) and 1986 (○)

160

pody, ophthalmology and physiotherapy — that patients often fail to utilise in other settings[14,52]. They also have organised recreational activities, holidays and outings, and spacious and well set out grounds tempting to developers. Despite the prejudicial connotations of a "total institution", these activities take place in a vital, ongoing community, with caring staff, from porters and telephonists to cooks, who are tuned to patients' idiosyncracies and needs, and under constant peer and external scrutiny.

In planning for the care of hospitalised psychotic patients, who are at present being looked after in units that provide an asylum from wanton cruelty and neglect, little thought is being given to those very ill patients who are not being looked after anywhere at all — and it is surely these patients who should be our first priority, instead of reorganising our services to meet the articulate demands of the least needful, under the guise of bold and imaginative planning.

Acknowledgement

Some of this chapter has been adapted from material collected for a forthcoming book, *Community Care and Psychiatric Rehabilitation*, due for publication by Baillière Tindall in 1988, in which proposals are made for the development of community provisions.

I thank Dr J. Taylor for an interesting talk on the early history and the librarians of Friern Hospital for their help.

References

1. Sprenger, J. and Krämer, H. (1487). *Malleus Maleficarum* or *The Witch Hammer*. Translation by Summers, M. (1971), p. 482. Arrow Books
2. Report of the Select Committee on Criminal and Pauper Lunatics (1807), p. 4
3. Report of the Metropolitan Commissioners in Lunancy (1844), p. 92
4. Wing, J. K. and Brown, G. W. (1970). *Institutionalism and Schizophrenia*. London: Cambridge University Press
5. Weller, M. P. I. and Heager, B. *Psychiatric Rehabilitation and Community Care: Three Cases.* (Submitted for publication)

6. Tooth, G. C. and Brooke, E. M. (1961). Trends in the mental hospital population and their effect on future planning. *Lancet*, **1**, 710–13

7. Editorial (1961). *Lancet*, **i**, 1151

8. Waind, A. P. B. (1961). Needs and beds. *Lancet*, **i**, 884 (letter)

9. DHSS (1981). *Care in the Community: A Consultative Document on Moving Resources for Care in England*. London: DHSS

10. Egan, G. P. (1961). Needs and beds (letter). *Lancet*, **i**, 1284–5

11. Farris, R. E. L. and Dunham, H. W. (1939). *Mental Disorders in Urban Areas*, p. 134. Chicago: University of Chicago Press

12. Hollingshead, A. B. and Redlich, F. C. (1958). *Social Class and Mental Illness: A Community Study*. New York, London and Sydney: John Wiley

13. Royal College of General Practitioners (1981). *Survey of Primary Care in London*. Occasional Paper No. 16

14. Weller, B. G. A., Weller, M. P. I., Cocker, E. and Mohamed, S. (1987). Crisis at Christmas 1987. *Lancet*, **1**, 553–4

15. Heimler, E. (1967). *Mental Illness and Social Work*, p. 140. Harmondsworth and Victoria: Penguin

16. Warner, R. (1985). *Recovery from Schizophrenia: Psychiatry and Political Economy*. London, Boston and Henley: Routledge and Kegan Paul

17. North East Thames Regional Health Authority Report on Feasibility Studies, Appendix D.4, July 1983

18. Bosanquet, N. (1985). *Public Expenditure on the NHS: Recent Trends and the Outlook*. London: Institute of Health Services Management

19. Weller, M. P. I. (1985). A mental hospital's share. *Lancet*, **i**, 984–5

20. Goffman, E. (1961). *Asylums*. New York: Doubleday Anchor Books

21. Borus, J. F. (1984). Strangers bearing gifts: A retrospective look at the early years of community mental health centre consultation. *Am. J. Psychiat.*, **141**, 868–71

22. Donovan, C. M. (1982). Problems of psychiatric practice in community mental health centres. *Am. J. Psychiat.*, **139**, 456–60

23. Winslow, W. W. (1979). The changing role of psychiatrists in the

community mental health centres. *Am. J. Psychiat.*, **136**, 24–7

24. Benaim, S. (1983). The Italian experience. *Bull. Roy. Coll. Psychiat.*, **7**, 7–9

25. Raimon, S. (1983). Psychiatria democratica: A case study of an Italian community mental health service. *Int. J. Health Serv.*, **13**, 307–24

26. Hankin, J. and Oktay, J. S. (1979). *Mental Disorder and Primary Medical Care*. Rockville, Maryland: NIMH

27. Fink, P. J. and Weinstein, S. P. (1979). Whatever happened to psychiatry? The deprofessionalization of community mental health centres. *Am. J. Psychiat.*, **136**, 406–9

28. Clare, A. W. (1980). Community mental health centres. *J. Roy. Soc. Med.*, **73**, 75–6

29. Johnstone, E. C., Owens, D. G. C., Frith, C. D. and Calvert, L. M. (1985). Institutionalisation and the outcome of functional psychoses. *Br. J. Psychiat.*, **146**, 36–44

30. McCreadie, R. G., Robinson, A. D. T. and Wilson, A. O. A. (1985). The Scottish survey of new chronic in-patients: Two year follow-up. *Br. J. Psychiat.*, **147**, 637–40

31. Freeman, H. and Alpert, M. (1986). Prevalence of schizophrenia in an urban population. *Br. J. Psychiat.*, **149**, 603–11

32. Odegaard, O. (1932). Emigration and insanity: a study of mental diseases among the Norwegian born population of Minnesota. *Acta Psychiat. Scand.*, **Suppl. 4**, whole issue

33. Jauhar, R. and Weller, M. P. I. (1982). Psychiatric morbidity and time zone changes. A study of patients from Heathrow Airport. *Br. J. Psychiat.*, **140**, 231–5

34. Weller, M. P. I. and Jauhar, P. (1987). Wandering at Heathrow Airport. *Med. Sci. Law*, **27** (1), 37–9

35. Barclay, P. M. (Chairman) (1982). *Social Workers: Their Role and Tasks*. London: Bedford Square Press

36. GLC Health Panel (1983). *Mental Health Services in London*. London: Mind

37. Brahams, D. and Weller, M. P. I. (1985). Crime and homelessness among the mentally ill. *New Law J.*, **135**, 761–3; **135**, 626–9. Reprinted (1986) in *Medico-Legal J.*, **54**, 42–53

38. Martin, F. M. (1984). *Between the Acts: Community Mental Health*

Services 1959–1983. London: Nuffield Provincial Hospitals Trust
39. DHSS (1975). Cmnd 6233, *Better Services for the Mentally Ill*. London, HMSO
40. Martin, F. M. (1984). *Between the Acts: Community Mental Health Services 1959–1983*. London: Nuffield Provincial Hospitals Trust, p. 169
41. Cohen, N. L. (1984). The mentally ill; Homeless isolation and adaptation. *Hosp. Com. Psychiat.*, **35**, 922–4
42. MacKenzie, D. (1984). Italian madhouses. *New Scientist*, 30 August, p. 9
43. Jones, K. (1962). *Medical Care*, **1** (3), 160
44. Kraepelin, E. (1919). *Dementia Praecox*. Translation by Barclay, M. (Robertson, G. M., ed.), p. 34. Edinburgh: E & S Livingstone
45. Costall, B. and Naylor, R. J. (1986). Neurotransmitter hypothesis of schizophrenia. In Bradley, P. B. and Hirsch, S. R. (eds) *The Psychopharmacology and Treatment of Schizophrenia*, pp 132–65. Oxford, New York and Tokyo: Oxford University Press
46. Mueser, K. and Dysken, M. (1983). Narcotic antagonists in schizophrenia: a methodological review. *Schiz. Bull.*, **9**, 213–25
47. Tamminga, C., Tighe, P., Chase, T., Fraites, G. and Shaffer, M. (1981). Des-tyrosine-gamma-endorphin administration in chronic schizophrenics. *Arch. Gen. Psychiat.*, **38**, 167–8
48. Casey, D., Korsgaard, S., Gerlach, J., Jorgensen, W. and Summelsgaard, H. (1981). Effect of des-tyrosine-gamma- endorphin in tardive dyskinesia. *Arch. Gen. Psychiat.*, **38**, 158–60
49. Manchanda, R. and Hirsch, S. R. (1981). Des-tyr-gamma-endorphin in the treatment of schizophrenia. *Psychol. Med.*, **2**, 401–4
50. Verhoeven, W. M., van Praag, H. M., van Ree, J. M. and de Wied, D. (1979). Improvement of schizophrenic patients treated with [des-Tyr1]-gamma-endorphin (DT gammaE). *Arch. Gen. Psychiat.*, **36** (3), 294–8
51. van Ree, J. M., Verhoeven, W. M. and van Praag, H. M. (1980). Antipsychotic effect of gamma-type endorphins in schizophrenia. *Lancet*, **2**, 1363–5
52. Weller, B. G. A. and Weller, M. P. I. (1986). Health care in a destitute population: Christmas 1985. *Bull. Roy. Coll. Psychiat.*,

September, 223–5

53. Amdur, M. A. and Souchek, J. (1981). Death in aftercare. *Comp. Psychiat.*, **22**, 619–26
54. Haughland, G., Craig, T. J., Goodman, A. B. and Siegel, C. (1983). Mortality in the era of deinstitutionalization. *Am. J. Psychiat.*, **23**, 377–85
55. Sturt, E. (1983). Mortality in a cohort of long-term users of community psychiatric services. *Psychol. Med.*, **13**, 441–6
56. Roy, A. (1982). Suicide in chronic schizophrenia. *Br. J. Psychiat.*, **141**, 171–7
57. Pokorny, A. D. and Kaplan, H. B. (1976). Suicide following psychiatric hospitalization. *J. Nerv. Ment. Dis.*, **162**, 119–25
58. Scott, R., Gaskell, D. G. and Morrell, D. C. (1966). Patients who reside in common lodging houses. *Br. Med. J.*, **2**, 1561–4
59. Report from the research committee of the British Thoracic and Tuberculosis Association (1971). *Tubercle*, **52** (1), 1–18
60. Pinker, R. (1982). An alternative view. In Barclay, P. M. (chairman) Committee Report *Social Workers: Their Role and Tasks.* London: Bedford Square Press

Chapter 8

The evolution of the hospices

Dame Cicely Saunders

History inevitably includes something of the bias and experience of the person who is interpreting it and this account is given as my view of the roots and principles of the modern hospice movement.

St Christopher's Hospice, unlike nearly all the other modern hospices, grew into the local community rather than out of it. It developed from talks with patients, many of whom had pain from terminal malignancy, as their needs and achievements stimulated the ideas that gradually came together. Eventually St Christopher's was somewhat surprised to find that it had started a movement which has developed with a great variety of interpretations. The very first patient back in 1948 asked for "what is in your mind and in your heart" and I have always thought that meant all the skills that could be brought together with friendship for each individual person in pain. As he was dying with cancer of the rectum, with pain and vomiting and other symptoms, he knew he needed not only pain control but also personal concern. But there were other roots and many inputs along the way that I will try to describe briefly.

Figure 1 is a family tree, designed by Robert Twycross, our second research fellow at St Christopher's. My only comment is that there should be at least a dotted line from the Marie Curie Homes from which we certainly derived some ideas.

The original hospices go back further still to Fabiola, a Roman matron who opened her home for those in need in the early 4th century,

167

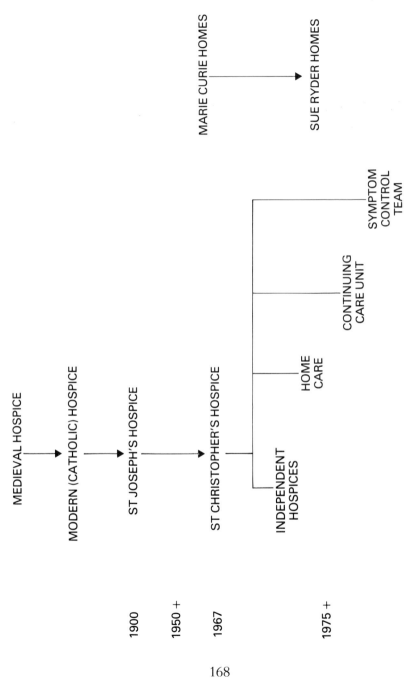

Figure 1 The development of hospice care (Reproduced from Reference 1)

168

setting out to fulfil the Christian "works of mercy": feeding the hungry and thirsty, visiting the sick and prisoners, clothing the naked and welcoming strangers. At that time the word "hospis" meant both host and guest, and the "hospitium" both the place where hospitality was given and also the relationships that arose. That emphasis is still central to hospice care today. From then on the church attempted to carry the burden of the poor and the sick and continued with this throughout the whole of the Middle Ages. In England this came to an abrupt end with the dissolution of the monasteries. None of these hospices set out specifically to care for the dying but they welcomed people to stay as long as they needed help, which must have included many who had care until they died. After the dissolution the state of those in need was sad indeed and many must have died at home in great poverty.

The first institution I found using the word "hospice" especially for care of the dying was in France; it had been founded by Mme Jeanne Garnier who, after first visiting people dying of cancer in the back streets of Lyons, opened what she called both a hospice and a Calvaire. I have a rather idealised picture of this but from a later photograph it looked to suffer from the overcrowding which I sometimes found when I started visiting some of the homes from 1948 onwards.

In England the first use of the word "hospice" was by the Irish Sisters of Charity at St Joseph's in Hackney in 1905. Their founder, Mother Mary Aikenhead, had already opened their first such hospice for the dying in Dublin in 1879 but there was, apparently, no connection at all between her and Mme Garnier. Other homes were opened around the turn of the century, including St Columba's in 1885, the Hostel of God in 1892 and St Luke's Home for the Dying Poor in 1893. The last was the only one founded by a doctor, Dr Howard Barrett. Of all the homes (and there were others in the United Kingdom and in the United States), it certainly seems that Dr Barrett's was the most similar in principle to today's hospice, the most lively and full of a very particular and personal interest in the individual patient. Dr Barrett does not write of "the poor" or "the dying" but of each individual person and his desolate family left at home with no welfare state support. He left a wonderful series of Annual Reports but he only rarely mentioned the treatment of pain.

I went to St Luke's, by then with the title "Hospital", as a volunteer nurse in the evenings for seven years from 1948 onwards and, having become a doctor in order to look at the pain of terminal malignancy, arrived at St Joseph's in 1958. For the first time they had a full-time doctor who wanted to do some research or at least to monitor clinical practice. The first difference was the introduction of the regular giving of oral opioids — this I had first seen at St Luke's. They could trace this back to around 1935, soon after the Brompton Cocktail itself was produced.

When I arrived at St Joseph's I found that they were giving their drugs "as required" and that they were using injections rather than oral medication. Here, as elsewhere at that time, one saw people "earning their morphine", and it was wonderfully rewarding to introduce the simple and really obvious system of giving drugs to prevent pain happening — rather than to wait and give them once it had occurred. Here too there was the potential for developing ideas about the control of other symptoms, and also for looking at the other components of pain. But first of all I must salute the Sisters of St Joseph's and the compassionate matter-of-factness of their dedicated care. Together we began to develop the appropriate way of caring, showing that there could be a place for scientific medicine and nursing. We could illustrate an alternative approach to the contrast between active treatment for an illness (as if to cure it were still possible) or some form of legalised euthanasia. Figure 2 illustrates how terminal

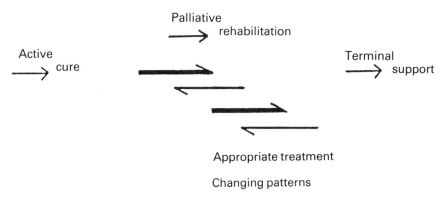

Figure 2   Appropriate treatment — changing patterns

care is part of a continuity of treatment, not a sudden soft option. Care and treatment should be given throughout, as we aim to enhance the patient's quality of life. As I looked at patients and could see, for example, the difference between a patient on admission full of the anxious tension of pain and the same person on his oral opioid, comfortably lying back able to complete his football pools, it gradually became apparent that here we had in fact reached a level of opioid dosage between the pain relief threshold and the sedation threshold.

Figure 3 shows that whether one starts with a smaller dose and increases slowly or with a higher dose and decreases it, the dose can be kept within the therapeutic band at the patient's own optimum dose. We found that the fears of drug dependence, of increasing tolerance or respiratory depression and even drowsiness were greatly exaggerated. We have since done a series of studies looking at this in detail, but with simple monitoring one was able to show that there was no escalation of dose, that one does not find the patient constantly asking for the next dose, that respiratory depression is not a clinical problem, and that in most cases any drowsiness wears off in about 48 hours.

However, it was more than the use of drugs. I remember one patient who said, when asked to describe her pain: "Well, doctor, it began in my back but now it seems that all of me is wrong," and she then

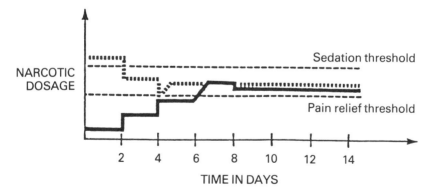

Figure 3 Alternative methods of dosage adjustment. Pain relief in the absence of sedation may be achieved with sequential increments in narcotic dose at intervals of 2 days (━━). In a few cases the severity of the pain will require an initially high dose, followed by sequential decrements until the pain reappears (■ ■ ■). A slight increase in dose provides analgesia without sedation (– – –). (Reproduced from Reference 3)

described her other symptoms. She went on, "I felt as if nobody understood me, all the world seemed against me. I could have cried for the pills and injections but I knew that I must not. My husband and son were wonderful but they were having to stay off work and lose their money." She was suffering a "total pain", and that is what we have been looking at over the years. It is, in a way, somewhat artificial thus to divide a whole experience but it may give an internal checklist on meeting a new patient. We saw, too, how important it could be to communicate something of the truth so that patients could take control of their own situation, and know that they were still in charge of themselves.

We began looking more closely at the family. They should not be together only for a celebration, or for just one or two visiting hours, and our concern should be with the whole group. This progressed to plans for home care. It was difficult to discharge people home when liaison was so poor and readmission complicated but I remember ringing up the family doctor of one patient (and that was not always easy). "We did very well," he said. "Did you push the diamorphine up much?" I asked. "No, but we pushed the whisky up a fair bit."

It seemed essential to found a new hospice where we could demonstrate all this and create an atmosphere in which those who were free of symptoms could search for meaning in their own way. Table 1 sums up the developments of the 1950s, when I was reading medicine, and the 1960s when I was at St Joseph's, gaining the hospice experience that was essential. Nearly all the psychotropic drugs were introduced during the 1950s, together with new non-steroidal anti-inflammatory agents and the synthetic steroids. There were now many new tools, adjuvants to the analgesics. There had been surveys and reports showing the need for better care, developments in palliative radiotherapy and oncology, the new pain clinics, and some work in home

Table 1 Developments in the 1950s and 1960s

1.	Hospice experience	5.	Pain clinics
2.	Clinical pharmacology	6.	Home care
3.	Surveys and reports	7.	Tavistock work on loss
4.	Palliative radiotherapy and oncology	8.	Theology and death

care which I had seen in both the United Kingdom and the USA. There was the Tavistock work on loss and bereavement to refer to and some writing on the theology of death. These came together in the design of the first modern hospice, bringing research and teaching into a unit with beds integrated into the community, with family care, a bereavement follow-up and a pioneer home care team. St Christopher's is unique in having also a residential wing for the elderly, with its priority for staff and their dependents and as a halfway house for a few patients.

Table 2 suggests possible hospice research projects. We have done a number of clinical series, including some backed by partial autopsies[3]. We have also tackled both studies in pharmacokinetics and double–blind controlled studies. These included a comparison of oral morphine and diamorphine, when it was found that given regularly with a phenothiazine there was no clinically observable difference. In 1977 we changed to using morphine as our standard opioid, and it now provides 80% of all the opioid doses given. It is important in any field to monitor clinical practice but especially so in an area that people are apt to think of as "a soft option".

One important study that we did, together with a pathologist and a surgeon from the Royal Marsden Hospital, looked at patients with, or without, salvage surgery for advanced head and neck cancer. There was no difference in the symptoms arising or in their control during the terminal phase, nor in length of survival. This is an important finding for those who are considering such surgery, particularly among elderly patients[4].

From 1974 onwards came the development of new ways of giving hospice care. St Christopher's had opened in 1967 and began home care two years later. I had been visiting groups in the United States from 1963 onwards and one of them launched the first hospice home

Table 2 Research in a hospice setting

1.	Case reports	5.	Clinical series
2.	Review literature	6.	Practice reports
3.	Statistics	7.	Pharmacokinetics
4.	Symptoms	8.	Controlled studies

care team with no back-up beds in Newhaven, Connecticut, in 1974. A doctor who had worked at St Christopher's and St Joseph's Hospice became their medical director and after a short time they enabled up to 70% of their patients to die in their own homes. Although ten years later they established their back-up beds, the American hospice pattern has been largely in home care, although not always with as much medical input as that Connecticut team. A Professor of Surgery came from Montreal for a sabbatical in the hospice and later opened a Palliative Care Unit in a teaching hospital. ("Hospice" in French Canada implies an alms house for the elderly.) He developed this special unit in 1975 as an integral part of the hospital, with its visiting teams consulting both in the hospital and in the home. The first of the UK Continuing Care units which were built by the National Society for Cancer Relief was opened in England at almost the same time and there are now a number of such units, fully part of the National Health Scheme. The final pattern, a consulting hospital team with no beds of its own, began its work in 1975 in a New York hospital. This second group had also been visiting with us. Multi-disciplinary teams have since developed in the UK, where St Thomas's set the pattern in 1978, and there are now over twenty in this country.

In many ways I think this is the most exciting way forward, helping to move support and symptom control to an earlier stage of disease. It emphasises that hospice treatment is not merely a last resort but can be practised in the general and teaching hospital. The discussion of problems over meals with contemporaries is, in fact, an important part of hospice development. Since 1967 there have been an increasing number of independent hospices and there are now over 2300 beds in this country. Most have their own home care teams or work with some of the over 400 "Macmillan" specialist nurses in the community. We can report increasing interest in the National Health Service as well. Improvement here is still patchy but special beds will always be few and our aim must be overall concern and education.

As we consider any hospice input to the problem of AIDS, let us not forget that some 140 000 people will die of cancer in the United Kingdom in any one year and more than half of them will have pain as a problem. It is only when such care is spread through the National Health Service in general, in both hospitals and the community, as well as in hospices, that these people will have the help they need. We have some evidence that pain control has improved in the hospitals near the hospice over a ten-year period but there is still a long way to go in our own field. We have knowledge to share but a heavy commitment to our own patients.

In summing up the elements of hospice care that have grown out of our historical roots and the great surge of development of the last twenty years in Table 3, I would still put symptom control first and emphasise that this calls for a team approach, whether it be by the clinical team, the nursing team, the interprofessional team or the home care team. We aim at maximising the potential that still remains for each patient and the family in the place of their own choice. This will be at home for as long as possible, but in some cases it will break down. Our concern then will still be with the patient and family together and what they can do with the time left to them. We aim to control symptoms in order to give a person freedom to move towards his own aims. Often this will be the resolution of family problems. People move fast in crisis and although the average length of stay in a hospice is only about three weeks, some can live a lifetime, or resolve longstanding problems, in that time. This makes all the difference for those who go on living afterwards, but there should be a bereavement service available for an identified minority. We have trained bereavement counsellors who are called in for about a quarter of the approximately 700 families we meet in a year.

Each hospice should consider suitable research and every unit or team will face a demand for its teaching, which may well include that of the general public. Approachable management is essential for good staff support which also calls for some kind of a community, rather

Table 3 Hospice care

1.	Symptom control	4.	Place of choice
2.	Teams	5.	Patient and family
	Clinical	6.	Bereavement service
	Nursing	7.	Management
	Interprofessional	8.	Community
	Home care	9.	Search for meaning
3.	Maximising potential		

more closely knit than an ordinary professional group of people enthusiastic about their job. We are all constantly challenged to a search for meaning with which to face both the questions that come from patients and family and the often draining demands of this work.

Figure 4 shows the many-headed dragon of terminal pain. This postcard was given to me by a patient saying, "That is what my illness feels like to me." It has to be tackled in detail and calls for constant review and follow-up, as we stay alongside. Figure 5 shows a second dragon, drawn by another patient during her last ten days to represent her illness. She has drawn herself as the child and although that dragon is eating up the flowers, the child is no longer afraid. Fear and apprehension are understandable — there is indeed a mystery ahead — but we can tackle fear of pain, fear of other symptoms, and, above all, fear of isolation. Although there will still be people who remain desolate or angry and with whom one has to wait alongside with no answers to give, the majority find their way into peace.

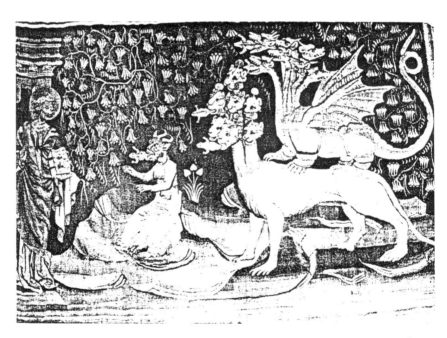

Figure 4   Tapestry de l'Apocalypse. Paris, 1380. (Reproduced from a postcard)

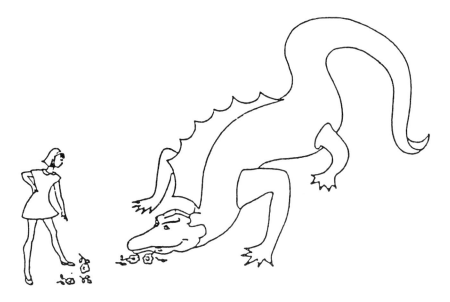

Figure 5   Drawing by Miss H. of her illness ten days before her death

Finally, we cannot ignore the fact that there is a spiritual dimension to this work. The longing for significance and meaning goes beyond our own capacity to fulfil but we can try to create an atmosphere in which others find a freedom to make their uniquely personal journey. Staff support here may best be found in the achievements made by many families, some of whom return years later. Hospice is still about relationships between persons and about their own reach to what they see as true. A free flying bird is a symbol used by many of the modern hospices. We make our own interpretations of this but with a common aim of helping all who come to have the freedom in which to make their own discoveries.

References

1. Twycross, R. G. (1980). Hospice care: redressing the balance in medicine. *J. Roy. Soc. Med.*, **73**, 475–81
2. Mount, B. M. (1978). Lecture given at the Annual Meeting of the

Royal College of Physicians and Surgeons of Canada, Vancouver, 27 January 1978

3. Baines, M. B., Oliver, D. J. and Carter, R. L. (1985). Medical management of intestinal obstruction in patients with advanced malignant disease. *Lancet*, **i**, 990–3
4. Pittam, M. R. (1982). Does unsuccessful salvage surgery modify the terminal course of patients with squamous carcinomas of head and neck? *Clin. Oncol.*, **8**, 195–200

Chapter 9

"The snowball effect": the growth of the treatment of intractable pain in postwar Britain

Jennifer Beinart

Intractable pain, that is, pain associated with a physical cause which cannot be cured or for which no physical cause can be found, remained one of the grey areas of medicine until well after the Second World War. In conditions ranging from terminal cancer to facial neuralgias or phantom limb pain, inadequate pain relief could present a major problem to many patients. Doctors from various specialties took an interest in the theoretical aspects and the treatment of such pain, but advances were limited. Although access to effective treatment of intractable pain is still uneven, there have been significant changes in the past thirty or forty years. These include drug innovations, theoretical advances, and new techniques. Equally important has been the discernible trend towards the provision of an institutional focus for such treatment: the pain clinic. This chapter aims to separate out these strands in an attempt to explain this growth. First, however, a word of explanation about the title.

My interest in the history of pain clinics and the treatment of in-tractable pain sprang from research into the history of anaesthesia, and, in particular, the history of one department of anaesthesia during the past fifty years. In interviews and in a questionnaire sent out to former members of the department, I asked people to give their reasons for choosing the specialty of anaesthesia. One respondent mentioned an interest in the phenomena of consciousness and unconsciousness; most said that they saw opportunities in the specialty for combining technical and scientific interests and for finding openings in a specialty that was clearly expanding after the war. Only one person mentioned an interest in "people, not putting them to sleep" — and he had not stayed in mainstream anaesthesia. This was John Lloyd, who worked in a pain clinic in Oxford in the early 1960s. He described (personal communication, 4 June, 1984) the "snowball effect" as word got around among doctors that someone was interested in pain, and more and more patients were referred to him for diagnosis and treatment. It seemed that the more he treated, the more kept coming; it grew like a snowball rolling downhill. The great problem that he had to contend with for many years was lack of beds — these were not his patients — and it was the struggle over this issue that led to a successful resolution in the establishment of an eight-bed Pain Relief Unit at Abingdon, near Oxford. Here, too, the number of patients has increased in a similarly spectacular way.

The "snowball effect" in the growth of the numbers of patients has been paralleled by a second such effect: the growth of a sub-specialty[1]. Its institutional form is the pain clinic, and the number of these has increased from zero in the 1950s to well over two hundred now. This is reflected in a professional association known as the Intractable Pain Society, founded in 1967 with seventeen members, and expanding exponentially to about four hundred now[2]. Although there has been much discussion about inter- or multi-disciplinary pain clinics, the great majority of members of the Intractable Pain Society are anaesthetists. Increasingly now, advertisements for posts in anaesthesia carry a suggestion that an interest in pain treatment would be welcome. It would seem, then, that the treatment of intractable pain has grown as a sub-specialty of anaesthesia. This is not to deny the important role of specialists from other fields both in treatment and in research; neurologists, in particular, have a long historical interest, especially in the theoretical aspects of intractable pain. Nor would it be correct to characterise anaesthetists as unanimous regarding the desirability of this sub-specialty. Some have argued quite forcefully that good management of intractable pain at the level of primary care would serve the patient's interests better, and would be far more cost-effective than the consumption of time and resources under specialists in hospitals[3]. However, those who hold such views are probably in a minority.

One explanation for the growth in pain treatment is the diffusionist model, which sees a pioneering example as the beginning which is followed by subsequent developments. This is part of the case presented by Steven Brena[4], in a survey of pain clinics around the world. He sees John Bonica's pain clinic in Seattle (founded on Bonica's reckoning in 1946) as a sort of beacon to which other would-be practitioners came to light the torch with which to establish pain clinics for their own countries. Another interesting strand of his argument concerns the growth of pain clinics in Western countries and the lack of such facilities in developing countries. Brena attributes this aspect of the global North/South divide to the greater longevity of more affluent peoples, leading to a greater incidence of low back pain.

One might argue that this is putting the theoretical cart before the horse. Firstly, as will be shown, in Britain at least, intractable pain treatment has grown up initially in association with the pain of terminal cancer, with some exceptions. Only when the institutional base was firmly established did other types of chronic pain come in on a large scale. Of course, the rise in cancer during this century may be associated with an increased average life span, but it seems doubtful whether this can be linked directly to the rise in intractable pain treatment. This leads to a second problem with Brena's argument. There has been no organised attempt to meet a perceived need for the treatment of intractable pain with a suitable service, on a national scale, in any of the advanced industrial countries. It appears rather that individuals have built such opportunities in a variety of ways, in the interstices of other more established specialist services. Pain relief is growing, but remained for a long time a low priority field. In poorer countries such a low priority subject simply does not receive any funding. It is poverty, not a lack of low back or any other type of pain, that would preclude the growth of pain clinics in less developed countries.

If the diffusionist model is not adequate, it is worth considering other types of explanation for the development of a hitherto neglected field in medicine. Most studies of professionalisation have dealt with non-medical subjects, but there are a few notable exceptions[5]. The issues are often very complex, and it is only by deliberately over-simplifying that a few factors are selected here, in order to provide alternative models. Firstly, there may have been a technical or drug innovation — the discovery of radium and the growth of radiology represent such a case. Secondly, there may be a rise in demand for treatment, from the consumers, or a recognition by doctors or public health experts that a great need exists — rising concern over cancer and the growth of oncology are examples of this. Thirdly, and per-haps the most difficult to identify, is the formation of a group of practitioners interested in providing a service, conducting research and so on, in a field which may have been neglected or of low status previously. The development of ophthalmology, for example, may be seen partly in these terms.

Most of the early work on chronic pain treatment in Britain centred on severe pain associated with terminal cancer. A precursor of some significance is a brief 1936 paper by W. Ritchie Russell[6], a neurologist at Edinburgh, on intraspinal injection of alcohol for intractable pain, in which he cited Dogliotti as his main inspiration. Alcohol continued to be used, but it carried a high risk of complications, particularly neuritis, which made it unattractive even in terminal cases. The idea seems to have been kept alive in the USA: J. R. J. Beddard[7], an anaesthetist who worked at Bath, described using intraspinal alcohol after reading an article published in an American journal in 1950. He had little success, because of difficulties with the catheter becoming curled in the spinal canal. Roger Bryce-Smith, an Oxford anaesthetist, also confirmed (personal communication, 4 July, 1984) that alcohol was not successful in sufficient cases to warrant wider use. He had been called in by Ritchie Russell, who was working in Oxford after the war, to try to treat patients with phantom limb and other types of pain. As in other instances, a neurologist called in an anaesthetist to place the needles in the hope that some kind of regional or spinal block would help his patients. Bryce-Smith found that very little seemed to help for very long, until the advent of a new and more promising approach. This was the intrathecal phenol technique pioneered by R. M. Maher[8], a physician at Rochdale. In a 1955 paper in *Lancet*, he described how the alternative agent, combined with a carrying solution that was heavier than the cerebrospinal fluid, made it possible to target the posterior nerve roots, which carried sensation from the painful areas, more accurately. As Maher put it, comparing his phenol in glycerin with the alcohol employed previously: "It is easier to lay a carpet than to paper a ceiling."

However, whilst a number of subsequent reports acknowledge the debt owed to Maher, some practitioners continued to use the nerve block techniques developed by Bonica and others, employing newer agents such as lignocaine. For example, an anaesthetist and a physician[9] at the Whittington Hospital in London published a report on the first hundred cases at their "pain clinic" in 1957, with no reference to Maher. Most significant among their references was probably the 1953 book by Bonica[10], entitled *The Management of Pain*. This massive tome was eventually to find its way onto the shelves of many British anaesthetists and others interested in the treatment of chronic pain.

Meanwhile, the traffic across the Atlantic was not entirely one-way. A multi-authored paper[11] in the *New England Journal of Medicine* in 1962 opened with a mention of Maher and the amplification of his work by Nathan and Scott of Queen's Square. One of the authors — they were all at Massachusetts General Hospital and Harvard Medical School and were mainly neurosurgeons — sent an offprint to Maher, with a note saying: "To Dr Maher, with great appreciation for your pioneer work in this field and gratitude for showing it to me. James C. White."

When the Oxford anaesthetist John Lloyd became involved in the pain clinic set up by Ritchie Russell in the early 1960s, it was run by a triumvirate of a neurologist, a psychiatrist and an anaesthetist. The others faded away gently, leaving the anaesthetist with his needles and solutions, which seemed at last to be hitting the spot. One reason they did so, apart from the hyperbaric phenol solution, was the time that this particular doctor was prepared to spend with patients, and the fact that he conveyed a belief in their suffering. He found that more and more patients were referred to him, some for whom he could do nothing. The cancer patients, for whom he generally could do something, were treated sometimes in their homes (as Maher had often done) and sometimes in hospital, so that the effects of an intrathecal injection could be monitored overnight. Beds had to be begged and borrowed, and when the pressure built up to impossible proportions the answer came, unexpectedly, from the Regional Hospital Board. Under a phase of reorganisation of resources there was spare capacity in a local hospital, which was channelled to Lloyd for what was designated a pilot study of terminal care.

In fact, from its opening in 1970 the Pain Relief Unit was a centre for the treatment of intractable pain. At first this was mainly cancer pain, but as referrals again snowballed, the greatest increase was in other types of pain, especially low back pain. New techniques, including cryoanalgesia, were evolved in the Unit, visitors from around the world flocked to see Lloyd and his team at work, and drug companies vied to sponsor research. Increasingly, this has been oriented towards the opioid drugs rather than to new ways of using needles for nerve blocks[12].

Both locally and nationally, the "snowball effect" has shown that there was no shortage of demand: once some provision had been made for the treatment of intractable pain, the demand appeared to be insatiable. What was the role of a new technique? In this case, for this country, I have singled out Maher's intrathecal phenol. It seems that it helped to give some practitioners the confidence to launch into this new, rather difficult area, in which few rules had been mapped out and in which they had to work with patients whom other doctors had not managed to help. The involvement of anaesthetists, still in the 1950s a marginalised group within the profession, is well explained in the words of one of them, who commented that this work "leads the anaesthetist away from his stool in the theatre to the bedside".

It is interesting, too, that so many of the earliest pain clinics were established in non-teaching hospitals in the provinces; this is another aspect of the marginality of this field. In the Oxford case I have referred to, the spectacular success story of the establishment of the first National Health Service unit for the treatment of intractable pain came about in a very convoluted way, almost it seemed by accident. And pain relief, an unknown quantity, had to masquerade as something more established in order to be accepted as needing beds — as terminal care (though this was itself still fairly marginal). It would seem, then, that the growth of the treatment of intractable pain in postwar Britain can be explained by the interaction of factors — technique, patient demand and practitioner demand — all operating in the gaps between established interests and services.

Finally, I would like to pay tribute to Maher for including as evidence of the usefulness of his technique photographs of some of his patients before and after treatment[13]. They were mainly middle-aged or elderly women with cancer, quite humble women in pinafores who were able to get on with the rest of their lives once the pain had been removed. In some cases, a patient was able to get back to work. That was not the most important effect of treatment, however. The smiles on these people's faces were in his view the best argument for making better provision for treating intractable pain.

References

1. Beinart, J. (1985). Pain relief — a new sub-specialty? *Bull. Soc. Social Hist. Med.*, **36**, 10–13
2. Swerdlow, M. (1983). The history of the IPS — Part 1. *IPS Forum*, **1**, 2–3. (See also: Nash, T. P., letter to author, 25 Sept., 1984. *IPS Handbook*, 1984)
3. Dwyer, B. (1983). Recent trends in pain clinics. *Anaesth. Intens. Care*, **11**, 54–5
4. Brena, S. (1985). Pain clinics around the world: an overview. *Clinics in Anaesth.*, **3** (1), 75–81
5. See for example: Larkin, G. V. (1983). *Occupational Monopoly and Modern Medicine*. London: Tavistock
6. Russell, W. R. (1936). Intraspinal injection of alcohol for intractable pain. *Lancet*, **2**, 595
7. Beddard, J. R. J. (1958). Twenty years of clinical nerve blocking. *Br. J. Anaesth.*, **30**, 367–72
8. Maher, R. M. (1955). Relief of pain in incurable cancer. *Lancet*, **1**, 18–20
9. Belam, O. H. and Dobney, G. H. (1957). Persistent pain. Treat-

ment by nerve block. *Anaesthesia*, **12** (3), 345–51

10. Bonica, J. J. (1953). *The Management of Pain*. London: Henry Kimpton

11. Mark, V. H., White, J. C., Zervas, N. T., Ervin, F. R. and Richardson, E. P. (1962). Intrathecal use of phenol for the relief of chronic severe pain. *N. Engl. J. Med.*, **267**, 589–93

12. Beinart, J. (1987). *A History of the Nuffield Department of Anaesthetics, Oxford, 1937–1987*, pp 123–32. Oxford: Oxford University Press

13. Maher, R. M. (1975). Cancer pain in relation to nursing care. *Nursing Times*, **71**, 344–50

Chapter 10

The management of obstetric pain

Wendy Savage

In writing on this subject I should like to pay tribute to Jennifer Beinart[1], of Oxford, and Donald Moir[2], the Glasgow anaesthetist, both of whom have written informatively about obstetric analgesia.

One must wonder whether obstetric pain is quite the right term, as each childbirth is different. It is clear that some women find childbirth extremely painful but other women do not seem to find labour painful. They may even enjoy labour. Even within the same woman, a first labour may be quite different from a second or a third labour: in one the woman may seem to have unbearable pain but in another it may be quite tolerable. This may be because of the way the baby is lying, it may be because it is a bigger baby, or it may be because of the atmosphere where she is actually labouring. If one looks at different groups and at different periods of history (or at different times in the same culture), one sees that labour has been dealt with in different ways by different cultures.

There is a model in which birth is a female celebration and the woman is supported by other women who have had children, older women. An atmosphere of gaiety pervades the whole labour. There are other times when the whole way that labour is approached seems to be punitive and the attitude of the midwife can then be absolutely crucial. The way a woman views her labour can resemble the way that pain can be experienced during war, for example. There are well documented occasions where people have not been aware of major injuries until after the battle was over — showing that there is a very important psychological component to the way pain is experienced. Also, there is a difference in the way that women labour at home, in familiar surroundings, compared with the way that they labour in a modern labour ward, which is not a cosy, quiet and relaxed place, and where the woman may be surrounded by strangers. This does perhaps raise the question whether the psychological state of the woman affects the way she labours. How otherwise does one explain the enormous rise in Caesarean sections that has taken place in most Western countries (but not all), from 4.5% in both this country and the USA in 1970 to just over 11% in this country and 24% in the USA in 1985. One cannot believe that this is all to do with the attitude of the obstetrician. One cannot believe that the human race would have overpopulated itself to the extent that it has, if it were necessary for one woman in four to be delivered by Caesarean section. American studies[3] on the increasing Caesarean section rate suggest that one of the biggest causes for the operation has been dystocia, difficult labour — and this despite the probability that the population is more healthy than it has ever been before. Something else seems to be going on besides the fear of litigation, and the interventionist attitude of obstetricians. There is something also going on in women and I think one of the things that is happening is that women are losing their confidence in their ability to deliver their babies normally.

Much of the traditional attitude towards pain in childbirth seems to be based on the statement in Genesis: "In sorrow you shall bring forth children." Sir James Young Simpson was one of the people who questioned, a hundred and forty years ago, whether this was, in fact, a correct translation because, after all, this is an English translation of a Greek translation of something that was written in Hebrew. In the *New English Bible* the same passage has been translated somewhat differently: "I will increase your labour and your groaning and in labour you shall bear children." Now that seems to me to be much nearer to the truth. The idea that the woman is allowed, encouraged even, to express her feelings by vocalising is, I think, another of those areas where the modern labour ward has changed in the thrall of anaesthetists who are keen on epidural anaesthetics and who say how nice and quiet the labour ward is. Well, should the labour ward be quiet? I have never forgotten going to deliver a Turkish woman when I was a medical student on the district. When we were two blocks away on our bicycles we could hear the rhythmic rise and fall of her wails. Everybody was there supporting her and she had a very easy delivery. She was absolutely delighted — and it was part of the way that labour was approached. In contrast, the sound of an Indian patient that I also had when I was a student and who was squatting in the corner of the corridor of a barren ward in the hospital, crying with each contraction, separated from the women who would have supported her in her own country, surrounded by people who didn't even speak her language, showed that this was an altogether lonely and terrifying experience for her.

The different attitudes that we can have are well expressed by this quotation from Doris Lessing's *A Proper Marriage*[4], which was written in the 1960s but, I think, probably relates to her own experience of childbirth before that:

> "It was a pain so violent that it was no longer pain, but a condition of being. The wave receded however, just as she decided she would disintegrate under it. She went limp, into a state of perfect painlessness, in which the mere idea of pain seemed impossible."

This is now the second stage of labour:

> "The room was full of people again. She was sucking in chloroform like an addict and no longer even remembered that she had been determined to see the child born."

The women quoted in *Spiritual Midwifery*[5] — a book written by Ina May Gaskin, who in the 1970s taught herself to be a midwife in Tennessee, in a community known as the Farm — did not even use the words "pain" and "contraction". They talked about "rushes". This is one woman's description of her labour:

> "Even now I have not been rushing I was still opening up. I was 8 cm. It broke my water bag and I had several nice

strong rushes and was ready to push. It felt really good to push. I felt the baby slide under my bones and start up the birth canal. Doctor Gene rubbed baby oil on and massaged my muscles. He felt as tantric and loving as one of the other midwives, he is really a gentle man. I was very grateful to have him help me. Once I got the baby through the bones, I had to slow down a little. Finally out popped his head. I panted, no cord. I pushed again. It is a boy, a beautiful, healthy baby boy. He weighed 8 lbs, even though he was a month early. Donald and I have big babies. It was nice to have a boy. We already had two girls. I had not torn. It was the first homebirthing Doctor Gene had ever done. He was amazed, really amazed. He was really glad he had done it. He had had a really good time. We all did. "

Last year I took part in a television programme for Granada. An obstetrician on the panel said that he thought that it was nonsense when women said that they could enjoy labour. I was delighted when a general practitioner obstetrician in the audience, a man, very quiet and bespectacled and not at all a flag-waving sort of person, said how saddened he was that an obstetrician who had reached retirement had done so without understanding that women could enjoy labour. He had learnt this when he started to do home deliveries; and although he had not been particularly in favour of this idea, as he was able to give women the choice he had now a large practice of women having home deliveries and had learnt from that how women behave.

The history of obstetric analgesia suggests that up to five thousand years ago various societies used opiates or herbs, or counter-irritants. A nice example is given by Moir[2] of how in one Samoan group the man sits behind the woman and when she has a contraction he pushes his heels into her ribs as a good counter-irritant. It is interesting that although acupuncture has been used by the Chinese for so long, it has rarely been used in childbirth to control pain, although there is an acupuncture point. When I visited China last year, I was told that Chinese women are strong, they don't need any help with the pain. My guide said that many of her generation, who were women who were deferring having the only child they were going to have until they were in their thirties, were actually seeking places where they could have a Caesarean section because they were so frightened of the pain. And yet, China, in the 1950s, because of its closeness to Russia used psychoprophylaxis. However, the political climate has changed and now psychoprophylaxis is no longer the right thing for Chinese women to do. Consequently, they have no pain relief. Because of the American influence they deliver their babies in the lithotomy position, just like American women, but without the caudal or epidural anaesthetics that American women would be given.

The history of analgesia in the UK began with Sir James Young Simpson who, in January 1847, a mere three months after ether had been used for the first time, tried it on a pregnant woman. He then tried out chloroform later in that same year. A few years later Queen Victoria made chloroform respectable, at least for the upper and middle classes, by having it in her own childbearing. After seven without it, one feels she was perhaps entitled to have a little whiff of the gas! However, many people thundered against the use of chloroform, saying that women were supposed to suffer, that they would not love their children if they had not felt the pains of labour, that it was necessary for women to feel pain, and that it was in some way protective. There was not, of course, any evidence at all to substantiate this. I have certainly met women who, because of those terrible days in the 1950s when sometimes women would labour for three days before they gave birth, never really felt they loved their children because of the pain that they had suffered in bringing them into the world. "One child infertility", where women never have another pregnancy because of their fear of labour pain, designates a group of women that I remember well, but I think that this condition has disappeared now that we have the ability to help relieve pain in those women who need help.

Klikovitch, in St Petersburg in 1880 tried out nitrous oxide, and then Karl Gauss in Germany in 1903 started using twilight sleep. With this technique, using morphine and scopalamine, the woman had no recollection whatsoever of the labour and woke up to find the baby lying next to her in the bed. Jennifer Beinart[1] has pointed out the very interesting fact that feminists in the United States were fighting for twilight sleep to give them more control over themselves, rather than losing control during unanaesthetised labour, until the death of Mrs Frances Carmody, in Long Island in 1915, reduced the popularity of the method. However, in the UK some people were using this method right up to the 1930s, and in some parts of the USA it is used to date!

It was in the 1930s that the National Birthday Trust Fund launched a fund for analgesia for poor women and this finally culminated in the introduction of the Minnitt Gas and Air Machine, which was designed by a Liverpool anaesthetist in 1933. The machine was approved by the Central Midwives Board in 1936. It is interesting that in the same year that the machine was developed, 1933, Grantley Dick Read wrote his first book, entitled *Natural Childbirth*[6]. This was based on his observation of women of non-English cultures who seemed to give birth without the pain that he had been used to seeing women suffer when he was a medical student at the London Hospital. That book dropped without trace and nobody took any notice of it. In 1942 he wrote a second book, called *The Revelation of Childbirth*[7], in which he went further into his theory that the pain of labour was due to fear leading to tension and therefore to pain, and that if the fear were removed women could have a painless labour. It was re-issued in the United States with the title *Childbirth without Fear*[8], the title that most people know him for. This was the situation as World War II approached. In 1939, despite the Central Midwives Board approval of the Minnitt machine, only 29 out of 188 local authorities had midwives trained in the use of nitrous oxide. The vast majority of women before the Second World War therefore did not have a chance to use this method. During the mid-20th century there was a great growth, particularly in the USA, of the use, which had begun in Germany, of spinal, epidural and caudal analgesia for women in labour and especially women in the second stage of labour. The details of the development of the use of spinal and then caudal anaesthesia are of great interest, though beyond the scope of this review.

The reason that the Central Midwives Board and the National Birthday Trust were particularly interested in volatile anaesthetics was that they wanted something that was safe to use at home. Chloroform, which was used by doctors at home, was not considered safe for midwives to use. It is interesting that trichloroethylene, or Trilene, was first used in 1941 and fourteen years later was approved for use by midwives. Penthrane was used widely in the United States in 1959 but never really became established in the UK, although by 1970 midwives in Wales were allowed to use it.

Pethidine, which, of course, is the mainstay of treatment in the UK, was not synthesised until 1939. It was first used for women in labour in Germany, but the war intervened and it was not until much later that it was used in England.

There have been three national surveys of births in England and Wales. The first was carried out in 1946 by Douglas[9], the second was undertaken in 1958[10] and the third was completed in 1970[11] (see Figure 1). In 1946 over 60% of women had no analgesia at all. At this time 46% of women had their babies at home and the Caesarean section rate was 1%. 16% of women used gas and air and 17.5% used chloroform. There was a small group of 4.6% who had a mixture of various agents. Pethidine did not rate a mention in 1946 because the war had prevented access to the relevant information.

By 1958 the proportion having no analgesia had dropped to 22.2%. The number having gas and air was 53.5% By then a mixture of nitrous oxide and oxygen was used by 0.3%. Many of the Minnitt machines seem in fact to have delivered a lot of nitrous oxide and not very much oxygen and it may be that the pain was relieved because the woman was so anoxic. However, the babies did not seem to do any worse than with other methods of analgesia according to the 1958 survey. Trilene was relatively popular at 22.6% and chloroform was no longer used at all. In 1970 the way the questions were asked was somewhat different. Only 2.7% used no analgesia, but it is possible that one should add the 18% who had no analgesia because of the use of pudendal block. By this time only 2% were using gas and air, but 52% were using gas and oxygen. 7.1% were using Trilene.

According to the same surveys, as shown in Figure 2, pethidine was not used in 1946, a few women had opiates and mixtures but there were no epidural anaesthetics, although in the United States epidurals were quite commonly used. In 1958 54.5% had pethidine. By 1970, 68.9% of women had pethidine, another 5% had other opiates, and epidurals appear for the first time, 0.9%. In that survey 0.1% of women used hypnosis and about 5% used psychoprophylaxis — that was 269 women out of the 16 000. Of these women, as the

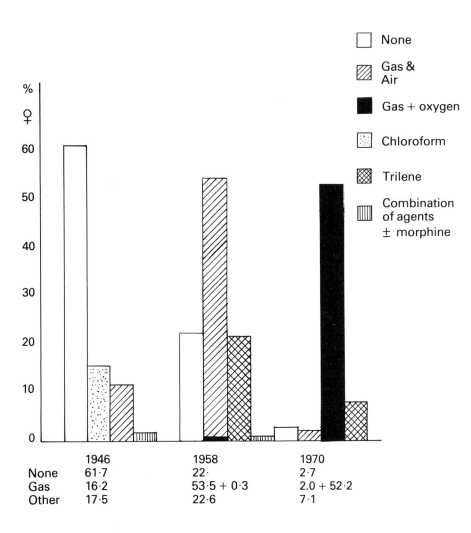

Figure 1 National surveys on the use of inhalational anaesthesia in England and Wales

authors point out, only 12% using psychoprophylaxis used nothing else; that is, it did not sound markedly effective as a method. When one looks at this change in the pattern of use, the question of whether so many women do need to be using analgesia does arise, as quite a lot of women have relatively quick labours. Even allowing for the 1.0% who had paracervical block or other regional anaesthesia, I would have thought that more than one woman in five would be able to go through labour without any analgesia.

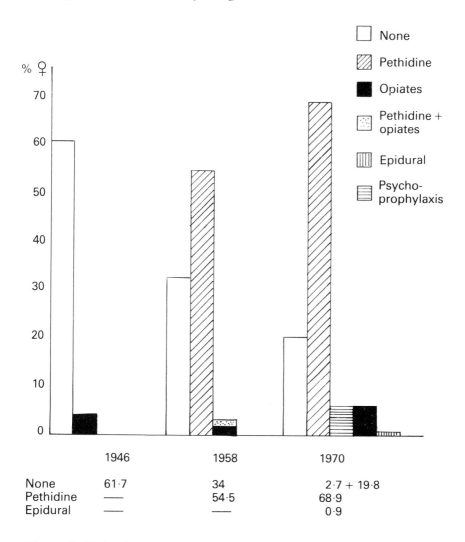

Figure 2 National surveys on the use of non-inhalational forms of analgesia in England and Wales

The attitude of staff or the influence of the climate in which the woman delivers is, I think, well shown in Table 1, which compares the use of obstetric analgesia in the London Hospital and Queen Charlotte's Hospital[12] in 1981. In the latter only 8% of women had no analgesia, whereas in the London Hospital almost 50% had no analgesia. There the Asian patients tend to be multiparous women and they tend to come in later, but it is interesting that the relatively low percentage of women using analgesia is not because of the Asian women, who, if anything, used analgesia slightly more. A mixture of gas and oxygen was used by slightly more at the London Hospital than at Queen Charlotte's — and pethidine slightly more again, but that is because of the very different rate of use of epidural analgesia. Half of the women at Queen Charlotte's at that time had an epidural analgesic, while at the London Hospital only about 7% did so. The figures for Queen Charlotte's do not mention general anaesthetic at all and, of course, some of the patients at the London Hospital who had a general anaesthetic may have had no analgesia before that, but some may have had pethidine, and this might influence these numbers a little.

It does seem extraordinary that just about seven miles across a major capital city can make so much difference in the use of analgesia. What is it about the London Hospital that makes it have very low proportions of women using analgesia compared with probably most other teaching hospitals in Britain at this time? It is not that its facilities

Table 1 Obstetric analgesics in two London teaching hospitals in 1981

	Queen Charlotte's Hospital (%)	The London Hospital	
		Caucasian patients (%)	Asian patients (%)
None	8	47.2	42.0
Gas and oxygen	12.8	16.4	19.5
Pethidine	20.8	27.9	31.6
Epidural	42.3 } 50.8	8.5	6.9
Epidural and other	8.5		
Miscellaneous	5.2	} 21.1	13.3
Pudental block	2.4		
General anaesthetic		11.5	13.0

196

are completely inadequate. It is true that there is no epidural service and it is true that the epidural rate is down to 3%. But in the 1950s Mr Perchard, as a young consultant, introduced the use of hypnosis into the London Hospital, Mile End, and midwives were trained to continue that tradition. Of course the computer form does not note the use of hypnosis, but some of the women who were recorded as having no analgesic were actually using this self-hypnosis technique. I think that the attitude of the midwives and the consultant obstetricians has a great deal to do with the way that a woman is offered pain relief. I myself realised that my attitude was wrong when I was working in Professor Morris's unit in 1976. I went to see a woman who was having her first baby, and she seemed to me to be making rather heavy weather of it. I said to her, "I think it would be a good idea if you had some pethidine." She said, "I don't want any pethidine, thank you," to which I replied, "Well, I have seen far more labours than you have and my advice to you is to have some pethidine." That was a really heavy thing to say, I now realise. When I went to see her the next day, she said to me, "You know, you were quite wrong about that pethidine, because I felt that I was doing alright and I felt in control. When you said that to me I thought, 'Well, you must know,' but it really destroyed my ability to keep control of myself," and I realised that I had destroyed her whole feeling of her labour. Fortunately she forgave me and fortunately I learned from that experience. But I think that if you listen to what women say, you will find that many of them do not want to have the rhythm of their labour disturbed.

I was very struck when I saw a recent television programme on the Tower Hamlet midwives. In each of the two births shown, both of which were very calm, there was a point where the woman said, "I can't go on, it's too much," and each time different midwives said, "Yes, you can, we are all in it together." There was a definite feeling of female solidarity. It seemed to me that this is where the male obstetrician would say, "Well, would you like an epidural, would you like an injection?", because he does not take part in that feeling unless he has been supporting his own wife, perhaps, during a labour and he understands how much it means to her.

One of the motives for studying medicine is that the person wants to help people and unconsciously, I think, they have a greater fear of pain or disease than those who don't choose medicine as a career. Doctors want to do something to actually relieve pain. Because men seem more technically orientated than women, they want to do something about it that is technical, and maybe that is why they like the whole procedure of epidural analgesia. If one says to a woman that only four women out of five are going to have a perfectly acceptable level of pain relief by having it, that one woman in a hundred is likely to suffer a dural tap, which will leave her with a headache for five days and means she will have to lie flat on her back, that the actual injection may be fairly uncomfortable, and that the reported literature does give a 1 in 5000 risk of neurological damage (though the figures are perhaps better than that today), then how many women would actually *choose* to have an epidural? When a woman recently sustained a disaster at the time of an epidural in a nearby hospital, the demand for epidural analgesia fell smartly. Likewise, the demand also fell a few years ago when a woman at another hospital had a problem after a top-up.

My own view is that it is a wonderful anaesthetic when it works, when it is done by somebody who is properly trained, for women who have prolonged labour and who are likely to need some assistance with their delivery, and I think it is a splendid anaesthetic for doing Caesarean sections. I do not feel that more than 10–15% of women really need an epidural and the fact that in Holland 38% of women still have their babies at home and have no analgesia does, I think, show that it is not necessary for all women to be offered an epidural. One of the really difficult things is that if you have a service, then you have an anaesthetist whose job it is to give epidural anaesthetics. I see them prowling round the labour ward, looking for a likely candidate! And then they go to the relaxation classes or parent craft classes and they sell epidurals as this wonderful thing that leaves you absolutely in control, except you cannot feel anything, and you may not be able to pass urine and you cannot walk, but you are in control of yourself and you will be able to see your baby being born and feel no pain. It is a very difficult thing to set up a service that is there when you really want it, immediately, without it being oversold. This is the historical stage that we are at now, that we have anaesthetists who are beginning to say, as they did in a leading article[13] this year, that we must centralise deliveries so that we can have obstetric analgesia, given by anaesthetists, fully available — and this at a time when some obstetricians were perhaps beginning to think that maybe all this centralisation of deliveries wasn't such a wonderful idea after all.

I am left with the thought of McKinley that "the success of innovation has little to do with its intrinsic worth; that is, whether the innovation is measurably effective as determined by controlled experimentation, but dependant upon the power and level of interest that sponsor and maintain it." In England today we are seeing a big push for the pain of childbirth to be dealt with by a highly sophisticated, technical exercise — the giving of an epidural anaesthetic, but we have not spent anything like the same time and energy on helping women to prepare themselves for labour and to cope with it in the way that they want to. Dissatisfaction has been expressed by many women regarding the way that obstetrics is organised today. This became clear to me when I was suspended, through the letters that I received, and I think it is something that we, as a profession, need to address ourselves to. If one looks at the history of the management of pain in obstetrics it can be seen that there have been fashions in it ever since effective means to relieve pain became available, and these have led some cultures to use one method and other cultures to use another. But if women in Russia and women in France can learn behavioural techniques to help them to cope with the pain of labour, and if in some parts of Europe it is not even called the pain of labour even though contractions are felt which may sometimes be uncomfortable, it seems quite unnecessary for us to build great empires providing epidural anaesthetics for all, when there are so many people who do need pain relief in other areas. It is to these areas, such as in the management of intractable pain, that I think our resources need to be directed.

References

1. Beinart, J. (1986). *In Sorrow ..., Obstetric Analgesia and the Control of Childbirth in Twentieth Century Britain*. Oxford: Wellcome Unit for the History of Medicine. Unpublished monograph
2. Moir, D. D. and Thorburn, J. (1986). History of obstetric analgesia. In *Obstetric Anaesthesia and Analgesia*, 3rd edn, pp 1–8. England: Baillière Tindall

3. NIH Task Force (1981). Report on Caesarean section. Washington, USA: National Institutes of Health

4. Lessing, D. (1954). *A Proper Marriage*. Republished by Panther Books, London

5. Gaskin, I. M. (1977). *Spiritual Midwifery*, pp 72–4. USA: The Book Publishing Company

6. Read, G. D. (1933). *Natural Childbirth*. London: Heinemann

7. Read, G. D. (1942). *Revelation of Childbirth*. London: Heinemann

8. Read, G. D. (1944). *Childbirth without Fear*. London: Heinemann

9. Joint Committee of the Royal College of Obstetricians and Gynaecologists and the Population Investigation Committee (Douglas, J. W. B., ed.) (1948). *Maternity in Great Britain*. London: Oxford University Press

10. Butler, N. R. and Bonham, D. G. (eds) (1963). *Perinatal Mortality*. London: E & S Livingstone Ltd

11. *British Births, 1970*. A survey under the joint auspices of the National Birthday Trust Fund and the Royal College of Obstetricians and Gynaecologists, Vol. 2. London: Heinemann

12. Morgan, B., Bulpitt, C. J., Clifton, P. and Lewis, P. J. (1982). Effectiveness of pain relief in labour: survey of 1000 mothers. *Br. Med. J.*, **285**, 689–90

13. Reynolds, F. (1986). Obstetric anaesthetic services. *Br. Med. J.*, **293**, 403

Index

201

cancer
control of terminal pain of, 167, 170–5,
181–2, 184
role of endogenous opioids in, 134
captopril, 96
carbolic acid, 78
cardiovascular depression, 67, 71
childbirth, 187–99
chloroform, 64, 65, 191, 192, 193
circumcision, 17
Clinoral, 86
clitoridectomy, 17
consciousness, altered state of, 34–5, 36,
37, 39, 41–4
Continuing Care units, 174
co-trimoxazole, 96
curare, 65, 68–9
cyclopropane, 64, 65, 67

diclofenac, 85, 89, 90, 94
sodium, 96
diflunisal, 87, 89, 90, 94
Dolobid, 87
dosages
in terminal illness, 171
of early anodynes, 51–2, 55

efficacy of ancient remedies, 52–4
emetine, 10
enalapril maleate, 96
endorphins
identification of, 131–2
in fakir studies, 36
in hypnotic analgesia, 42
in stress-induced analgesia, 133–4
in trance-type rituals, 41
network of, 132–3
enflurane, 67, 68
enkephalins, 131–2, 134
ether, 63, 64, 65, 66, 67
ethnic differences in response to pain, 40
ethyl chloride, 64
etomidate, 71
exercise, physical and opioid system,
35–6

fakirs, performances by, 35–6
Feldene, 87

fenbufen, 89, 90, 94, 96, 115
adverse reactions profile, 104, 106–7
fenclofenac, 89, 91, 94
fenoprofen (Fenopron), 86, 87, 89, 90, 94
feprazone, 80–1, 89, 90, 91, 94
finger amputation, ritualistic, 17
fire–walking, 31–5
flufenamic acid, 85, 94
flurbiprofen, 86, 87, 89, 90, 94
fomentations, 56, 60
freezing, 20
Froben, 87

gas, stupefying, 22
gastrointestinal reactions to NSAIDs,
88–91, 97–114
"gate theory of pain", 44, 134

halothane, 65–7, 68
headache, 97–113
hemlock, 17
henbane, 17, 55
hepatitis, 65–6, 97–113
heroin, 130
hexobarbitone, 70
hook-hanging, 36–9
hospices, 167–77
in America, 173–4
St Christopher's, 167, 168, 173
St Joseph's, 168, 169, 170–2
St Luke's Home for the Dying Poor,
169–70
hyperpyrexia, malignant, 67
hypnosis, 22, 33, 34–5, 41–4, 193, 197

ibufenac, 94
ibuprofen, 86–7, 89, 90, 91, 94, 96
adverse reactions profile, 100–2
Indocid, 86
indomethacin, 86, 89, 94, 96
adverse reactions profile, 102–5
indoprofen, 89, 90, 91, 94, 95
inhalational agents, 64–8
instruments, early surgical, 22–3
intravenous anaesthetics, 70–2
isoflurane, 68

jaundice, 66, 97–113